In Loving Memory

Mrs Carole D. Elwell

Dr Wadie Kirollos and Mrs Dalal Mikhael

Mr Syed Mohamed Abdullah Al-Haddad

Mr Alwyn Bodkin

In Loving Memory

NEUROSURGERY

This new edition of *Neurosurgery: The Essential Guide to the Oral and Clinical Neurosurgical Exam* provides a concise and practical guidebook of the core knowledge and principles for the International and Intercollegiate FRCS Specialty Examination in Neurosurgery. It is a vital resource for the American Board of Neurological Surgery (ABNS) and other neurosurgical examinations around the world.

Written by neurosurgeons at the top of their field and based on new guidelines, this book takes students through how to succeed in the FRCS neurosurgery exams and provides an overview of crucial short and intermediate cases designed to mirror the exam's testing of a candidate's clinical knowledge, diagnostic acumen, investigation and interpretation, treatment options and taking consent.

Including 72 vital online revision flash cards, covering critical and diverse examination cases from trauma to paediatric spine exams, this edition also contains crucial guidance to Vivas on the following:

- Operative surgery and surgical anatomy
- Investigation of the neurosurgical patient
- The non-operative clinical practice of neurosurgery

This book is a must-read for candidates preparing for the final Intercollegiate Specialty Examination in Neurosurgery (UK), International FRCS Specialty Examination in Neurosurgery as well as the American, Canadian, European and Australasian exams. In addition to helping candidates pass their final exams, this book provides wonderful insight into Neurosurgery for Medical Students, Surgical Residents and Neurosurgical Consultants.

NEUROSURGERY
The Essential Guide to the Oral and Clinical Neurosurgical Exam

SECOND EDITION

Vivian A. Elwell
BA Hons, MA (Cantab.), MBBS, MRCS, FRCS (Neuro. Surg)

Ramez Kirollos
MBChB, MD, FRCS (Ed), FRCS (Eng), FRCS (Neuro. Surg), European Certificate of Neurosurgery

Syed Abdullah Al-Haddad
MB BCh BAO (NUI), MSc (Trauma), MRCS, FRCS (Neuro. Surg)

Peter Alwyn Bodkin
BSc Hons (Anatomical Sci), MBChB, FRCS (Neuro. Surg)

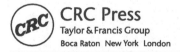

CRC Press
Taylor & Francis Group
Boca Raton   New York   London

CRC Press is an imprint of the
Taylor & Francis Group, an **informa** business

Second edition published 2023
by CRC Press
6000 Broken Sound Parkway NW, Suite 300, Boca Raton, FL 33487-2742

and by CRC Press
4 Park Square, Milton Park, Abingdon, Oxon, OX14 4RN

CRC Press is an imprint of Taylor & Francis Group, LLC

© 2023 Taylor & Francis Group, LLC

ISBN: 978-1-032-18405-0 (hbk)
ISBN: 978-1-032-13874-9 (pbk)
ISBN: 978-1-003-25437-9 (ebk)

DOI: 10.1201/9781003254379

Typeset in Utopia
by KnowledgeWorks Global Ltd.

Online Support Materials (Craven Flashcards) available at:
https://resourcecentre.routledge.com/books/9781032138749

Dedication

This book is dedicated to all healthcare staff for their responses to the COVID pandemic.

A certain excessiveness seems a necessary element in all greatness.

Harvey Cushing (1869–1939)

Contents

Foreword by Alistair Jenkins

Many years ago, I gave a talk at an international meeting on a particular procedure. I was feeling reasonably pleased with myself till one of my friends said to me afterwards, "You've never actually done that operation, have you...?"

You can always tell.

What you know is tested in the written part of a Neurosurgical exam. The Viva should test whether you know how to use this knowledge, and this excellent book repeatedly stresses the necessity of showing the examiner that you have performed or seen the common neurosurgical procedures, and can extrapolate sensibly from this experience to describe more esoteric operations.

I have another confession to make: Though I performed my first neurosurgical operation in 1981 and have been a UK Consultant for over 30 years, I have no formal neurosurgical qualification. When I trained, hours were very long and subspecialization rare. It was simply assumed that during your training you would absorb all you needed to know and could build on this as your career progressed. No formal testing was necessary or desirable.

In retrospect, this attitude could be described as both arrogant and ignorant. The randomness of both the chance of encountering enough cases of each condition and the interest and teaching ability of trainers meant I suspect that my generation ended up with frightening gaps in our knowledge – though on the positive side we did a lot more operating.

Since then, two things have happened: Around much of the world, and particularly in the UK, the working hours and thus clinical exposure of trainees have reduced considerably; and the sum of knowledge required has become considerably greater. In no field is the latter more apparent than in neuro-oncology: as well as mastering microsurgery, neuronavigation, 5-ALA, awake craniotomy and functional mapping, the aspiring neurosurgeon will need to be a pathologist, a molecular biologist, a radiologist – and a good communicator. When I was training? You took it out. Or didn't.

So in came exams, with the intention of ensuring that the successful candidate knew what was necessary to be a capable day one neurosurgeon. Not an expert, but safe and knowledgeable. While there is no way, short of direct observation, to assess actual operative skill, you are much more likely to be an effective surgeon if you know what you're talking about and can use that knowledge in a logical and sensible way.

This excellent book sets out to show you what you need, in almost every way imaginable, to pass an oral neurosurgery exam. It is written by examiners for candidates, and manages to get inside the minds of both to distill out the common problems and pitfalls; it then gives sensible and comprehensive ways for you to overcome these and – hopefully – pass.

Would I pass the Neurosurgery exit exam if I sit it tomorrow? Not a chance. But a few weeks with this book and I'd be well on my way – if I remembered not to pretend I had done operations I hadn't …

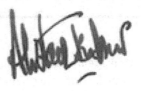

Mr. Alistair Jenkins, Consultant Neurosurgeon
Newcastle Hospitals NHS Foundation Trust, UK
Immediate Past President of Society of British Neurological
Surgeons (SBNS) 2022–2023

Foreword by John Pickard

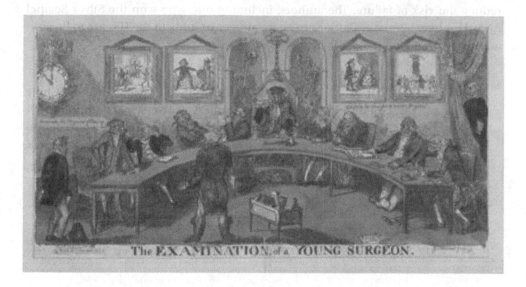

The EXAMINATION of a YOUNG SURGEON.

When I took the final FRCS in 1974, I had been working a 1:2 rota as a young registrar in general surgery, commuting from Glasgow to Falkirk. I had completed 18 months as SHO and Research Assistant in Neurosurgery with a first author paper in *Nature New Biology*. In London, the examiner asked me what specialty I wished to follow. On hearing that I was a fledgling neurosurgeon, he asked me to tell him what I knew about haemorrhoids.

> *'Plus ça change, plus c'est la même chose.'*

Two weeks later, I had better luck in Edinburgh. Shortly thereafter, I was on the plane to Philadelphia for my research fellowship. Stress, what stress.

Examinations are a necessary evil. Necessary because they provide an independent assurance to patients, families, the general public, employers, defence organizations, GMC, future colleagues, and all grades of staff that a successful candidate has acquired a basic core of knowledge and has displayed the ability to use it, albeit in the artificial environment of the examination hall. It is one important hurdle in the completion of training that indicates that the candidate is probably safe and has the flexibility of mind to cope with the ever-changing understanding of and technology within their specialty. 'Evil' because too many examinations and assessments can stultify, regiment thought and delay the development of lateral thinking and initiative.

However, like life, examinations can sometimes be unfair. As George Cruikshank's cartoon from 1811 illustrates, there was a time when examiners could be capricious in their judgement. There are now many checks and balances to reduce the risk of such errant behaviour. It is only right that examinations should be professionally organized and transparent in what is expected. Examinees in school and university have little else to think about. Trainee surgeons in their early 30s have patient care, research projects, families and mortgages to distract them.

There are occasions when an otherwise clinically competent candidate underperforms. This admirable and concise handbook provides invaluable insight and advice on how to prepare for the oral and clinical parts of Neurosurgery examinations and reduce the risk of failure. The authors, including one who won the Silver Scalpel Award for his many contributions to neurosurgery training in the UK, are to be congratulated on their initiative, insight and compassion.

Professor John Pickard CBE, FMedSci, FRCSEd, FRCS, MChair
Emeritus Professor of Neurosurgery, University of Cambridge UK
Former Chairman of Examiners, Intercollegiate Examination
in Surgical Neurology, UK

Preface to the Second Edition

Neurosurgery: The Essential Guide to the Oral and Clinical Neurosurgical Examination (Second Edition) provides a concise, logical and practical guidebook of the core knowledge and principles for the neurosurgical clinical exit examination.

You have demonstrated that you have the required knowledge by passing the written component of this examination. Your written knowledge must now be translated into an oral format in a safe, organized and confident manner. The main purpose of this 'exit' examination is to ensure that you are a safe and competent neurosurgeon.

Since the publication of the first edition of *Neurosurgery: The Essential Guide to the Oral and Clinical Neurosurgical Examination,* there have been major changes in many aspects of neurosurgical exam content, format and style. This reflects advances in current clinical practice as well as shifts in educational principles. The impact of COVID-19 has also had its effects on many aspects of life not least the delivery of neurosurgical exams. Some of these changes may be temporary but the ingenuity that had to be employed to maintain social distancing rules has been an opportunity to make the most of modern technology. It may well be that some of the lessons learnt will be continued in future exams.

Regarding advances in clinical practice, we have been particularly mindful of important subjects (e.g. increasing prominence of instrumentation in routine spinal work, changes in WHO grading of tumours, endoscopic techniques replacing the microscope in the anterior skull base, new scoring systems).

Although primarily designed to cover the UK exam, we recognize the increasingly global readership. We have now included many international exam formats as possible without diluting the intention of the original publication.

We continue to learn from teaching trainees at both the Aberdeen FRCS course and more recently at international courses for the International FRCS. Our interaction with trainees provides repeated opportunities to develop our understanding of how to get a trainee to maximize their potential in the exam. We provide ideas of the types of questions that may be asked and remain current on any changes in format. We cannot cover every aspect of exam preparation and there will always be an element of good or bad fortune on the day, but it is true that 'luck favours the prepared'. We hope this book helps and guides you with your preparation and the luck which comes along in equal measure!

Vivian A. Elwell
Ramez Kirollos
Syed Abdullah Al-Haddad
Peter Alwyn Bodkin

Acknowledgements

We would like to thank our colleagues, family and friends. This book would not have been possible without the ongoing support and encouragement of the following people:

Miss Elwell

The late Carole D. Elwell, Dr Nigel D. Mendoza, Miss Charlotte A. Mendoza

Mr and Mrs John A. Cervieri Jr., The late Carole D. Elwell, Dr Nigel D. Mendoza, Miss Charlotte A. Mendoza, Mr and Mrs John A. Cervieri Jr., Mr and Mrs Lawrence Flick, Mr and Mrs Stephen Cervieri, The van Trotensburg Family, The Carey-Carpenter Family, The Archer Family, Dr Sandra J Ginsberg, Dr Richard Katz and the late Mr Khai Lam.

Dr Kirollos

The inspiration of my late parents Dr Wadie Kirollos and Mrs Dalal Mikhael, the support of my wife Nivine and sons Karim and Sherif

Dr Al-Haddad

The late Mr Syed Mohamed Al-Haddad, Mrs Rabiah bt Othman, Munirah Aljoofre, Khadijah, Alwi, Zainab and Mohamed, Osman, Ading, Aman, Intan and Hussein Al-Haddad

Dr Bodkin

The encouragement (and cajoling) of my parents Alwyn and Norah Bodkin, the constant support of my wife Leeanne and our two children Jessica and Lewis

Authors

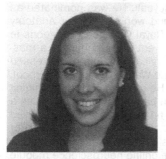

Vivian A. Elwell BA Hons, MA (Cantab.), MBBS, MRCS, FRCS (Neuro. Surg)

Having completed her specialist registrar neurosurgery run-through training and Post-CCT Senior Spinal Fellow in London, Miss Elwell is currently working as a Consultant Neurosurgeon and Spinal Surgeon at University Hospital Sussex NHS Foundation Trust. During her training, she has held posts in Accident and Emergency, Orthopaedics, Neurosurgery and General Surgery within the Surgical Rotation at St Mary's Hospital, Imperial College Healthcare NHS Trust, London. Miss Elwell's awards include the Swinford Edward Silver Medal Prize for her OSCE Examination; the Columbia University Research Fellowship at Columbia College of Physicians and Surgeons in New York City, USA; the Columbia University King's Crown Gold and Silver Medal Awards; the Kathrine Dulin Folger Cancer Research Fellowship and the 'Who's Who Young Scientists Award'. In 2010, Miss Elwell was a finalist for the BMA's Junior Doctor of the Year Award. She earned a bachelor's degree in biological sciences at Columbia College, Columbia University (New York City, USA) and a Master of Arts degree from the University of Cambridge. She earned a Bachelor of Medicine and a Bachelor of Surgery from the Imperial College School of Medicine. She is a Fellow of the Royal College of Surgeons.

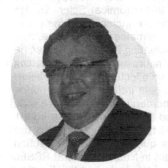

Ramez Kirollos MBChB, MD, FRCS (Ed), FRCS (Eng), FRCS (Neuro. Surg), European Certificate of Neurosurgery

In 1984, Dr Kirollos graduated from the Medical School at the University of Alexandria, Egypt. In 1987, he pursued his postgraduate medical education in the UK. He was awarded the Hallett prize by the Royal College of Surgeons of England for the results of his primary FRCS examination. Dr Kirollos trained in neurosurgery at the Atkinson Morley Hospital in London, the Frenchay Hospital in Bristol, the Leeds General Infirmary and the Walton Centre for Neurology and Neurosurgery in Liverpool. He obtained a Doctor of Medicine higher degree for his research into photodynamic therapy of pituitary adenomas. Dr Kirollos completed a skull base fellowship under Dr Gentili at the Toronto Western Hospital. In 2001, he was appointed Consultant Neurosurgeon at Addenbrooke's Hospital in Cambridge. In June 2018, Dr Kirollos moved to Singapore. His main clinical interests include anterior and middle skull base, pituitary and pineal surgery, and surgical treatment of arteriovenous malformations. A passion for neurosurgical technique based on the thorough understanding of anatomy has accompanied Dr Kirollos' neurosurgical training and forms the basis of his surgical practice. He keenly shares this philosophy and knowledge with his trainees. Dr Kirollos has been actively involved in day-to-day teaching of medical students and junior and middle-grade neurosurgical trainees. He has served on the faculty for Neuroanatomy of Operative Approaches and the British Neurosurgical Trainee courses since their conception in 2005 and 2010, respectively. In 2006, he was elected as a member of the Court of Examiners of the Royal College of Surgeons of England. In 2010, for his commitment to surgical education, he received the prestigious Silver Scalpel Award. He was in the past Chairman of the British Neurovascular Group (2013–2015), President and co-founder of the British-Irish Meningioma Society, member of the postgraduate educational committee of the EANS, ex officio member of the SBNS council as representative for the SBNS to the EANS and WFNS and currently is a member of the Neuro-Oncology Committee of the WFNS. Dr Kirollos has over 100 publications, 100 presentations and 50 invited lectures and is the co-editor of the *Oxford Textbook of Neurosurgery*.

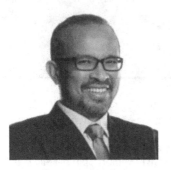

Syed Abdullah Al-Haddad MB BCh BAO (NUI), MSc (Trauma), MRCS, FRCS (Neuro. Surg)

Dr Al-Haddad is originally from Malaysia, where he studied and won the Most Outstanding Student Award from the Royal Military College. Subsequently, he was awarded a full scholarship to study medicine in the UK. During his undergraduate years, he excelled in both academic and extracurricular activities. He represented his college at the intervarsity level in rugby, hockey and volleyball. He was nominated as the sportsman of the year and won the Barker Anatomy Prize. He graduated from the Royal College of Surgeons in Ireland in 1996. In 2000, he went on to complete a master's degree at the University of Birmingham in the study of surgical outcome of depressed skull fractures. He commenced his neurosurgical training at the Walton Centre in Liverpool, where he developed his interest in neuro-oncology research. He undertook further training in neurosurgery in Manchester, Leeds, Aberdeen and Edinburgh before being appointed as a Consultant Neurosurgeon in Aberdeen, Scotland. Throughout, he has been actively involved in teaching both undergraduate and postgraduate students. He is a faculty member for Leeds and Edinburgh operative neuroanatomy courses. He has published numerous articles in peer-reviewed journals and also contributed a section to the online neuroscience module (www.ebrainjnc.com). Dr Al-Haddad is the Founder and Director of the highly successful Aberdeen FRCS (SN) Viva course. The course has run twice a year since 2010, with the emphasis on giving practical advice to produce outstanding neurosurgeons who are well prepared for the challenge of the neurosurgical exam.

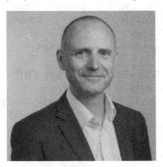

Peter Alwyn Bodkin BSc Hons (Anatomical Sci), MBChB, FRCS (Neuro. Surg)

Dr Bodkin grew up in Belfast and moved to Manchester for his medical degree. Whilst there, he took the opportunity of doing an Intercalated BSc in Anatomical Sciences. He reconstructed the facial features of ancient Egyptian mummies for his BSc project and has remained keenly interested in anatomy ever since. After graduating from Manchester, he went on to work in a number of neurosurgical units including Cambridge and Edinburgh. He was a lecturer and spine fellow at the Royal College of Surgeons in Ireland before embarking on his consultant post in Aberdeen. He maintains a wide breadth of surgical interests particularly in complex spine and facial pain. He was instrumental in setting up the Scottish National Teaching programme for Neurosurgery; he is the Chairman of the Scottish Neurosurgical Training Committee, a question writer for Section One FRCS (NS) exam, a member of the Surgical Specialty Board in Neurosurgery at RCSEd and Clinical Lead for Neurosurgery in Aberdeen. He teaches widely including the Surgical Approaches to the Spine Course in Edinburgh as well as his own course, the Aberdeen White Matter Tract Dissection Course. In addition, Dr Bodkin is responsible for the running of the Aberdeen FRCS (Neuro. Surg) Viva Preparation course.

Contributors

Professor Nabeel S Alshafai
Consultant Neurosurgeon
Nabeel S. Alshafai Neurospine Centre
Bahrain
Introduction

Mr Nicholas DP Hall
Consultant Neurosurgeon
Epworth Neurosciences Clinical Institute
Melbourne
Introduction

Mr Sohail Majeed
Neurosurgical Registrar
Aberdeen Royal Infirmary
Introduction
International FRCS

Mr Bedansh Roy Chaudhary
Consultant Spinal Consultant
Oxford University Hospitals NHS
    Foundation Trust
Chapter 1: How to Succeed

Mr Ioannis Tsonis
Neurosurgical Registrar
Aberdeen Royal Infirmary
*Chapter 2: Clinical Intermediate and Short
    Cases—Paediatric Examination*

Mr Phil Copley
Neurosurgical Registrar
Aberdeen Royal Infirmary
*Chapter 4: The Viva: Investigation of the
    Neurosurgical Patient—Paediatric
    Short Case*

Dr Charles Fry
Registrar in Neurophysiology
The Newcastle Upon Tyne Hospitals NHS
    Foundation Trust
*Chapter 4: The Viva: Investigation of the
    Neurosurgical Patient*

Mr Ravi Vashu
Consultant Neurosurgeon
Ampang, Malaysia
*Chapter 4: The Viva: Investigation of the
    Neurosurgical Patient*

Mr Khandkar Ali Kawsar
Consultant Neurosurgeon
The Royal Infirmatory of Edinburgh
Chapter 7: Landmark Publications

Miss Claudia L. Craven
Paediatric Spinal Fellow
Great Ormond Street Hospital
    Foundation Trust
London
Craven Flashcards

Examination Cases
Craven Flash Cards

Created by Claudia Craven, these 72 examination flash cards provide an invaluable revision resource for the final Intercollegiate Specialty Examination in Neurosurgery (UK), International FRCS Specialty Examination in Neurosurgery as well as American, Canadian, European and Australasian exams.

All 72 flash cards can be accessed at:

https://resourcecentre.routledge.com/books/9781032138749

- ☐ Examination Cases
- ☐ General and Trauma
- ☐ Brain-Stem Death
- ☐ Mental State Examination
- ☐ Speech and language
- ☐ Upper Cranial Nerves
- ☐ Lower Cranial Nerves
- ☐ Oncology and Epilepsy
- ☐ Frontal lobe
- ☐ Temporal lobe
- ☐ Parietal lobe
- ☐ Occipital lobe
- ☐ Surface Anatomy
- ☐ Cerebellar Examination
- ☐ Seizure Examination
- ☐ NF1
- ☐ NF2
- ☐ Tuberous sclerosis
- ☐ Von Hippel–Lindau
- ☐ Sturge–Weber (Encephalotrigeminal angiomatosis)
- ☐ HHT
- ☐ Skull Base and Pituitary
- ☐ CP Angle (Cn 5,7,8 + cerebellum +/- hearing and consider NF2)
- ☐ Nystagmus
- ☐ Hearing Examination (Cn 8)
- ☐ Cushing's Examination
- ☐ Acromegaly Examination

Note: Memorise the House-Brackman Score

- ☐ Vascular
- ☐ Anatomy of brainstem
- ☐ Stroke syndromes
- ☐ Wallenberg/Lateral Medullary
- ☐ Delayed cerebral ischemia
- ☐ Eye and CCF Examination (Cn2,3,4,6 and 5)

Note: For AVM – Examine the Appropriate Lobe

- ☐ Fundoscopy
- ☐ Functional
- ☐ Autonomic Dysfunction
- ☐ Face Examination (Horner's syndrome, MG, Cn5 and Cn7)
- ☐ Trigeminal Dermatomes
- ☐ Hands and Tremor Examination
- ☐ Parkinson's
- ☐ Coordination (Cn8, Cerebellar, PD)
- ☐ Spine
- ☐ Gait Examination
- ☐ Back Examination
- ☐ Sensation
- ☐ Arms/Upper Limb Examination
- ☐ Lower Limb Examination
- ☐ Peripheral Nerve
- ☐ Pathways of Nerves
- ☐ Pathways of Nerves

- Ulnar nerve
- Median nerve
- Median nerve
- Radial nerve
- Hand exam
- Thoracic Outlet Syndrome
- Foot Drop Exam
- Cerebrospinal Fluid
- Adult Shunt Exam (IIH, Hydro)
- NPH Exam
- Syringomyelia and Chiari Exam
- Paediatric

- Paediatric Developmental Examination
- Paediatric Head Examination
- Lambdoid vs. Positional
- Paediatric Shunt Examination
- Paediatric Pineal Examination
- Paediatric Spine Examination
- Paediatric Gait Examination
- Operations To Know
- Operative Complications
- Viva Topics Draw or Interpret

Example: Speech

	Test [2 mins]	Looking for	Key Anatomy
☐ Ask	☐ Intro – Wash Hands, Right / Left / Profession ☐ Can I look at your neck?	☐ Spontaneous and fluent speech ☐ Scars tracheotomy or ACDF	
☐ Speech	☐ Please cough and say "eeeeee" ☐ Say yellow lorry, baby hippotamus ☐ Count 1–10	☐ Dysphonia ☐ Dysarthria ☐ Pace (cerebellar – rush) and Volume (PD)	☐ Timbre – Superior Laryngeal n. ☐ Hoarse – Cricothyoird – RLN ☐ Lower cranial nerves – Velum
☐ Language	☐ Repeat this sentence (cow jump over moon) [stand behind them] follow instruction (paper) ☐ Name these 3 objects ☐ Repeat: Car, Key, Train	☐ Fluency and understanding ☐ Understanding ☐ Word finding – nominal ☐ Repetition	
☐ Summary	☐ Thank you. In summary: ☐ Speech: Spontaneous Speech: No dysphonia or dysarthria and good pace, good volume ☐ Language: Fluent, intact comprehension, word- finding intact and able to repeat	☐ Global aphasia – both Broca + Wernicke ☐ Wernicke – Fluent (meaningless), poor compression, and can't repeat [Transcortical sensory same but can repeat]. ☐ Broca – Expressive – non-fluent, compression intact, can't repeat [Transcortical motor same but can repeat] ☐ Conductive – can't repeat ☐ Anomia – pure word finding	☐ Broca + Wernicke ☐ W – Angular gyrus BA 40/22 ☐ B – Inferior frontal gyrus, Pars opercula. and triangul. BA 44 ☐ C – Supramarginal gyrus temporal lobe (Arcuate fasciculus)
☐ Complete	☐ Offer – Read this sentence and Write ☐ Full neuro examination, SLT assessment and flexible naso-endoscopy (dysphonia) ☐ MRI	☐ Dyslexia and Dysgraphia (confounders) ☐ Global aphasia, Wernicke, Broca, Transcortical Sensory or Motor, Conductive ☐ Dysarthria (spastic – from back of mouth, extrapyramidal – quiet, monotone, cerebellar – slurred, lower cranial nerve – nasal and breathy – 'D' difficult e.g. MG /bulbar) ☐ Dysphonia – Recurrent laryngeal nerve palsy, intubation, reflux	

Introduction
Getting Familiar with Exam Format

Every country has its own regulations around certification to allow for safe practice of neurosurgery, a major part being professional examinations. These can take many formats often involving some written elements and some more practical oral discussions. This book does not cover the written, knowledge-based components of the neurosurgical examination. Instead, we concentrate on the practical examinations that judge how a trainee applies their knowledge to real-life clinical situations, how they deal with stress, communication skills, clinical reasoning and professionalism. There will be slightly different emphasis according to each individual examining body. The British FRCS exam places particular value on gleaning a good crisp history, clinical examination, and clear management plan. In others, there will be more emphasis on how one performs surgical procedures or technical aspects. Some countries even expect surgical skills to be observed and assessed. We list below the formats of the major neurosurgical exam across English-speaking nations.

Intercollegiate Specialty Examination in Neurosurgery (UK and Ireland) – FRCS (Neurosurgery)

Postgraduate surgical exams in the UK and Ireland are conducted through the Royal Colleges of Surgeons (of Edinburgh, England, Glasgow and Ireland). After passing the Intercollegiate Membership of the Royal College of Surgeon examination (MRCS) in the early years of training, British trainees sit for the Fellowship exam (FRCS) in the final two years of specialist training. The Intercollegiate Surgical Curriculum provides the framework for neurosurgical training in the UK. It provides the neurosurgical syllabus and establishes the required standards for the completion of training. The Joint Committee on Intercollegiate Examinations (JCIE) regulates specialty fellowship examinations (jcie.org.uk). Section I of the exam is written, and Section II is the oral clinical component of the examination and consists of a series of carefully designed and structured interviews on clinical topics. Only after successful completion of Section I, candidates progress to Section II. Candidates have a maximum of 7 years to complete the two sections and up to four attempts to pass Section II. Section II is run twice a year at one of the neurosurgical units in the UK or Ireland. This exam takes place over two days.

Day 1 is for **Clinicals**, usually conducted within the local hospital complex. These comprise 'Intermediate Cases' and 'Short Cases'. Previously, candidates had one 'Long Case' over half an hour. Now there are two 20-minute **Intermediate Cases**.

For these, candidates will be asked to take a history (7 min) and examine (7 min) a patient, then present the examiner with their differential diagnosis, investigation plan, treatment options and potential complications (6 min). **Short Cases** comprise four 10-minute discussions in 40–minutes. Patients are not present for Short Cases. Instead, they are clinical scenarios testing categories such as: Clinical knowledge, Diagnostic acumen, Investigations and interpretation, Treatment options and Taking consent. The JCIE regulations state that 'Generic skills in information gathering and giving, professionalism and clinical conduct, structured approach and logical order, and clinical reasoning and judgement will also be assessed for Intermediate and Short Case Clinicals.'

Day 2 is for **Orals**. These cross-table exams are often held in a hotel or University/surgical College building. They comprise three 30-minute examinations covering: Operative Surgery and Surgical Anatomy; Investigation of the Neurosurgical Patient including Neuroradiology and the Non-operative Clinical Practice of Neurosurgery.

Examiners give a score from 4 to 8 for various aspects of the candidate's performance (see below). The candidate will need to average 6 and above to pass.

The FRCS exams are tightly regulated. Examiners convene several times a year to write new questions, review results of recent exams, standard set and update old questions. Very thorough statistical analysis is used to ensure that questions are at an appropriate level. Examiners are observed and assessed on their consistency and fairness. Most would agree that it is a fair exam with a realistic reflection of the day-to-day work of most neurosurgical consultants.

If you happen to do extremely well, you may be rewarded with the Norman Dott Medal. This award is given to a candidate who achieves the highest mark in the examination at the first attempt. The receivers of this award include the most highly regarded and eminent neurosurgeons of their generation. One is even included among the authors of this textbook!

In a series of workshops, Intercollegiate Surgical Board examiners identified nine aspects that they will assess in the oral examination.

1. Personal qualities, e.g. behaviour, attitudes, personality, honesty, integrity, demeanour.
2. Communication skills.
3. Professionalism.
4. Surgical experience and ability to integrate competencies.
5. Organization and logical, step-wise sequencing of the thought process; ability to focus on the answer quickly.
6. Ability to justify an answer with evidence from the literature.
7. Clinical reasoning, decision-making skills and prioritization.
8. Adaptability to stress and ability to handle stress.
9. Ability to deal with 'grey areas' in practice and complex issues that may not have been assessed by the other assessments.

JCIE Question Review Checklist for Oral Question Writing

Question Review Checklist

Alignment	Is the task required by the question congruent with the tasks required of a Day One consultant in the generality of the specialty?
Higher order questions	Are all the questions associated with the scenario 'Higher order' questions (i.e. questions which require candidates to think rather than simply remember facts; see *Example higher order questions*)?
Open questions	Are the questions open-ended to invite discussion rather than single-phrase answers?
Level of competence	Is the question pitched at the right level to discriminate between candidates either side of the level of the Day One Consultant?
Jargon	Is the question jargon free (as much possible within the topic area)? Is it free from idioms which might unfairly disadvantage non-native English speakers?
Timing	Can examiners and candidates do justice to the question within the time allocated for each Oral question?
Clarity	Is it clear from the question what candidates are expected to do?
Window dressing	Is all the information in the scenario and associated images useful for answering the question? Questions which can be answered without referring to the scenario or images are typically pitched at the recall level. They also use up precious time in the examination by giving candidates irrelevant information to process.
Marking	Does the question elicit the skills listed in the JCIE Marking Descriptors? Is it possible to score a 4? Is it possible to score an 8?

The Official Scoring Sheet Provided by the Examination Board – Intercollegiate Specialty Board Marking Descriptors

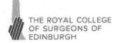 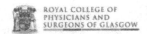

THE ROYAL COLLEGE OF SURGEONS OF EDINBURGH

Royal College of Surgeons of England

ROYAL COLLEGE OF PHYSICIANS AND SURGEONS OF GLASGOW

RCSI

Joint Committee on Intercollegiate Examinations

Marking Descriptors

Rating Scale	Overall Professional Capability / Patient Care					Knowledge and Judgement			Quality of Response		"Bedside Manner"
	Personal qualities	Professionalism and ethics	Surgical experience	Adaptability to stress	Ability to deal with grey areas	Knowledge	Ability to justify	Clinical reasoning	Communication skills	Organisation and logical thought process	Applicable to Clinicals with patients
4	• The candidate demonstrated incompetence in the diagnosis and clinical management of patients to a level which caused serious concerns to the examiner					• Did not get beyond default questions • Failed in most/all competencies • Poor basic knowledge/judgement/ understanding to a level of concern • Serious lack of knowledge			• Q: Does not get beyond default questions • A: Disorganised/confused/ inconsistent answers, lacking insight • P: Un-persuadable – prompts do not work		• Abrupt/brusque manner • Arrogant • Inappropriate attitude/behaviour • No empathy • Rough handling of patients • Totally inappropriate examination of either sex
5	• The candidate failed to demonstrate competence in the diagnosis and clinical management of patients					• Demonstrated a lack of understanding • Difficulty in prioritising • Gaps in knowledge • Poor deductive skills • Poor higher order thinking • Significant errors • Struggled to apply knowledge/ judgement/ management • Variable performance			• Q: Frequent use of default questions • A: Confused/disorganised answers; hesitant and indecisive • P: Required frequent prompting		• Does not listen-patronising • No introduction • Unsympathetic • Unobservant of body language • Inappropriate examination of either sex
6	• The candidate demonstrated competence and confidence in the diagnosis and clinical management of patients					• Competent knowledge and judgement of common problems • Essential points mentioned • Instils confidence • No major errors • Logical approach to difficult problems			• Q: Answers competence questions correctly • A: Methodical approach to answers; has insight • P: Requires minimal prompting		• Appropriate introduction • Appropriate examination of either sex • Considerate examination • Shows respect • Responds to patient/ carer
7	• The candidate demonstrated ability and confidence above the level of competence					• Ability to prioritise • Comfortable with difficult problems • Good decision making/demonstrated good level of Higher Order Thinking/ provided supporting evidence and familiar with literature			• Q: Answers difficult questions correctly • A: Demonstrates clear thinking process to difficult questions and answers. • P: Fluent responses without prompting		• Gains patient confidence quickly • Good awareness of patient's reaction • Puts patient at ease quickly
8	• The candidate demonstrated ability and confidence very significantly above the level of competence					• At ease with higher order thinking • Flawless knowledge plus insight and judgement • Had an understanding of the breadth and depth of the topic, and quoted from literature • High flyer • Strong interpretation/judgement			• Q: Stretches examiners – answers questions at advanced level • A: Confident, clear, logical and focused answers • P: No prompting necessary		• Exceptional communication/ relationship with patient/ carer

JCIE/Marking/Marking Descriptors Jan 2013   [Q: questions A: answers P: prompting]

Joint Committee on Intercollegiate Examinations
Policy No. G38 v1.0

International FRCS Exam (Neurosurgery) – JSCFE

The Joint Surgical Colleges' Fellowship Examination (JSCFE) is a relatively recent qualification offered by the four Royal Surgical Colleges (England, Edinburgh, Glasgow and Ireland) to the international surgical community.

On passing the JSCFE, you will be awarded the international qualification FRCS (College) and are eligible to apply for election as a Fellow to any of the four Royal Colleges. You will then be entitled to use the colleges' associated postnominal FRCS (College). On completion of FRCS International, you are exempted from PLAB to apply for GMC general registration.

The exam assesses at the standard of the UK and Ireland fellowship examinations — applicants are therefore required to provide verification that this level has been reached in their training and/or clinical experience prior to sitting the exam. The supporting endorsement are normally provided by the trainers or senior colleagues. The final decision on eligibility for admission to the exam lies with the JCFE Subcommittee.

Regulations

1. Applicants must be 6 years medically qualified.
2. Applicants would normally have passed the MRCS examination of one of the four Surgical Royal Colleges, but this is currently not mandatory.
3. Applicants must have successfully completed a locally recognized surgical training programme and are required to provide evidence of having achieved the required standard of a recognized specialist (day 1 NHS UK/Ireland consultant standard) in the generality of Neurosurgery.
4. This evidence must consist of **three** structured references as follows:
   The **principal referee** must be the applicant's current of Head of Department or Head of the Recognised Training Committee/Programme in which the applicant has participated. The **second referee** must be a senior clinician who has worked with the applicant and has knowledge of the applicant's work in their specialty within the last 2 years. The **third referee** must be a senior clinician who has worked with the applicant and has knowledge of the applicant's work in their specialty within the last 2 years.
5. The final decision on eligibility for admission to the examination will lie with the Intercollegiate Specialty Board in Neurosurgery.
6. Examination attempts candidates have up to a maximum of 7 years to complete the examination process as follows:
   Section 1: Candidates will have a maximum of four attempts with no re-entry.
   Section 2: Candidates will have a maximum of four attempts with no re-entry.

Scope and format

Section 1 is a written test composed of two single best answer papers

Candidates must meet the required standard in Section 1 in order to gain eligibility to proceed to Section 2.

Paper 1: 120 Single Best Answer (SBA) (2 hours 15 minutes)
Paper 2: 120 Single Best Answer (SBA) (2 hours 15 minutes)

Section 2 is the clinical component of the examination

It consists of a series of carefully designed and structured scenario-based interviews on clinical topics – some being scenario based and some being patient based.

Clinical examinations

The Clinical Intermediate Cases – They are structured with approximately 5 minutes for history, examination and presentation of salient points, 5 minutes for interpretation of findings, differential diagnosis and investigation plan and 5 minutes for the treatment options and potential complications (two cases in 30 min).

The Clinical Short Cases – They will test categories such as: History taking and examination; Interpretation and differential diagnosis and Management plan/additional investigations and complications (four cases in 30 min). Generic assessment of information gathering and giving, professionalism and clinical conduct, structured approach and logical order and clinical reasoning and judgement will also be assessed for long and short cases.

Oral examinations

Three 30-minute orals in each of the following:

a. Operative surgery and surgical anatomy (30 min).
b. Investigation of the neurosurgical patient including neuro-radiology (30 min).
c. The non-operative clinical practice of neurosurgery (30 min).

Syllabus

The JSCFE syllabus defines the breadth and depth of knowledge, professionalism and clinical skills to be attained by surgeons in training. It specifies the levels of expertise to be anticipated at entry and at the various stages in training and defines the standards of competence expected on completion of the training programmes. The JSCFE adopts this standard as the one against which assessment will be made. The examination will assess various elements of applied knowledge, diagnostic skills, clinical judgment and professionalism.

Clinical management: The examination is set at the level of knowledge and standard required of a recognized specialist (day 1 NHS UK/Ireland consultant standard) in the generality of the specialty. Given the range of cases, the spectrum of complexity and the ability to deal with variations and complications within the practice of this specialty, a candidate should be able to demonstrate that their training/experience is such that they can safely manage both common and more complex clinical problems.

Operative skills: While the examination does not formally assess technical operating ability, the JSCFE considers it inappropriate to admit a candidate to the examination if there is any doubt as to their technical skills.

Professionalism and probity: The development of a mature and professional approach in clinical practice is essential for safe and successful patient care. Attitudes towards patients and colleagues, work ethic, ability to deal with stressful issues and the effectiveness of communication skills in providing supportive care for patients and their families are the professional qualities expected of successful candidates in this examination.

American Board of Neurological Surgery (ABNS)

This examination is composed of written and oral components. The oral exam comprises three sessions, each 45 minutes in length.

One session will be composed of five questions focused on general neurosurgery.

Topics include:

- Trauma craniotomy.
- Intracerebral haemorrhage (from any cause).
- Acute stroke care; hemicraniectomy, suboccipital decompression.
- Vascular dissection.
- Atherosclerotic vascular disease.
- Brain or spinal abscess.
- Intratumoral haemorrhage, pituitary apoplexy.
- Cauda equina syndrome.
- Spinal cord injury management.
- Spinal fracture management.
- Brain metastasis, adult glioblastoma, supratentorial meningioma.
- Hydrocephalus.
- Neurology (MS, temporal arteritis, other that mimics a surgical presentation).
- Baclofen pump failure, drug withdrawal/overdose.
- Peripheral nerve disorders.

One session will consist of five questions focused on the preidentified area of focused practice chosen by the candidate.

Spine
- Degenerative spine.
- Spinal tumours.
- Spinal vascular malformations.
- Spinal pain.
- Deformity.
- Instrumentation.

Tumour (Neuro-oncology)
- Glioma management.
- Brain metastases.
- Meningioma.
- Vestibular or other schwannoma.
- Brain mapping.
- Pineal region tumour.
- Intraventricular tumours.
- Spinal tumours.
- CNS lymphoma.
- Pituitary/sellar tumours.

- Endoscopic surgery.
- Skull base tumours.

Vascular

- SAH/aneurysm care (clipping, endovascular).
- AVM.
- AVF.
- Cavernous malformation.
- Ischemic disease/stroke.
- Endarterectomy.
- Bypass.
- Moya-Moya disease.

Functional

- Movement disorders.
- Epilepsy.
- Pain, trigeminal neuralgia.
- Behavioural disorders.
- Neurology (Parkinson's disease, Essential tremor).

Trauma/Critical Care

- Brain, spine, peripheral nerve injury surgery.
- Injury physiology.
- Critical care management.
- Intracranial pressure management.
- Secondary injury.
- Infection.
- Systemic injuries.

Paediatric Neurosurgery

- Full spectrum of cranial and spinal paediatric neurosurgery.

General

The candidate may choose a second general session of five cases.

Applicant cases' session

The third session will consist of five cases using case material submitted by the candidate.

- From the 125 cases submitted as part of the credentials review.
- Ten cases chosen for use at oral exam; five will be selected by the examiners for presentation by the candidate with discussion.
- Case data fields will generate a slide presentation for each case using ABNS software.

Royal College of Physicians and Surgeons of Canada

Unlike the ABNS, the RCPSC Board certification – also known as the Fellowship of the Royal College of Surgeons of Canada, FRCSC – of Canadian neurosurgical trainees takes place at the conclusion of the final year of the residency program. This examination comprises a 2-day written component, followed by a 1-day oral component.

FRCSC certification is a prerequisite for an independent neurosurgical practice in Canada. The focus is on the competency-by-design (CBD). The structure of the applied (oral) exam is six stations (20 min each), over 2 hours of evaluation.

Objective of the applied examination

The applied examination is designed to evaluate higher-order thought processes and clinical reasoning compared to knowledge and application of knowledge assessed in the written component. Stations can assess different and multiple CanMEDS roles (Medical Expert, Communicator, Professional, Health Advocate, Leader, Collaborator and Scholar). Examiners may interrupt the candidate to probe for answers, as well as to move the station forward so that the candidate is able to demonstrate their knowledge/clinical reasoning in the allotted time. Examiners may take notes during the stations and have been instructed to appear 'neutral' in their reaction to answers. They have been instructed not to provide feedback directly to the candidates. Observers may be present during some stations of the examination. These observers will not interact with the candidate or the examiners, or contribute to the candidate's scores in the station. They are there to observe the conduct of the examination process.

The format of the applied exam allows candidates to be examined by multiple examiners across a number of stations. For this reason, you may be examined by an examiner from your centre. Significant conflicts (e.g. a program director or mentor) are identified and avoided in scheduling your examination.

Content of the applied examination

The content of the examination is based on a blueprint that reflects the objectives of training in neurosurgery. The content is balanced to ensure an appropriate representation of the relevant domains. The applied examination may include stations that cover:

- Cranial.
- Vascular.
- Spine.
- Paediatric.
- Spine and peripheral.

Some of the issues that you may encounter in the exam include:

- Providing counselling through an ethical issue.
- Providing counselling regarding diagnosis, treatment, long-term management and prognosis.
- Demonstration or description of a focused physical examination.
- Obtaining a focused history.
- Visual recognition (laboratory reports, illustrations, scans).
- Videos.
- Critical appraisal.
- Structured oral encounters.
- Short verbal questions.
- How to come to a diagnosis.
- How to choose the appropriate care.

- How to prepare the patient, family and institution for the appropriate care.
- How to follow-up on the appropriate care.
- Technical aspects of care.
- Ethical issues.
- How to guide a patient/family through issues in a particular situation.
- A written clinical vignette (with or without images) followed by questions from the examiner including, but not limited to, discussions on diagnostic interventions, therapy and/or natural course of disease.
- Interpret videos, diagnostic imaging studies, laboratory investigations or results of other tests
- Interpret results of a physical examination.
- Demonstrate decision-making skills based on the case scenario and the interpretation of data.
- Provide a diagnosis and differential diagnosis.
- Demonstrate competency in communication with patients and health team members.
- Surgical management.
- Others.

Scoring of the applied examination

A global rating scale (GRS) will be used to assess relevant aspects of care demonstrated during the station. The GRS will be suited to the station and will focus on the candidate's ability to systematically work through a case, with a focused, rational and efficient approach.

The domains measured in the stations may vary, but most commonly include a selection from the following:

- Diagnosis.
- Clinical/patient management.
- Surgical maturity.
- Intrinsic CanMEDs roles – communication – e.g. clarity of expression, rapport building and/or information delivery/counselling skills.

Each station is weighted equally; station scores are combined and averaged to create an overall score for the applied examination.

European Association of Neurosurgical Societies

The oral examination is the second and final of the European Board Examination in Neurological Surgery. Successful candidates will be appointed as Fellow of the European Board of Neurological Surgery (FEBNS). The exam is open to those who meet all of the following criteria:

- Is an individual member of the EANS
- Has passed the Part I examination
- Has a Licence to practice neurosurgery (UK candidates are allowed to sit the exam in their final year of neurosurgical training if their training expires before the next year's exam)

It is a clinical problem solving and patient management test. It is not a theoretical examination, unlike the Part I examination. Case histories are given, and where appropriate, neuroimaging and other visual aids are shown to augment the presentation and development of cases. Candidates explain verbally how they would proceed to evaluate or manage the cases and to plan and perform the proposed operations, if indicated.

The examination, in the English language, consists of three parts, each lasting 30 minutes. Five to eight cases will be discussed during each part. Each of the three sessions is conducted in an interview setting with two examiners, experienced neurosurgeons from a European country. During these three sessions, the candidate will thus meet six different European examiners, each of whom will give an independent score. One session is dedicated to an oral examination on operative neurosurgery of the brain and skull. The other session covers operative neurosurgery of spine and cord. In the third session, the topics to be discussed will be those that could not be adequately covered in the first two sessions. A candidate who receives a passing grade for this examination will be granted FEBNS. If the Board finds that the quality of the best candidate's performance justifies this, they will be awarded the Braakman prize.

Indian Examinations in Neurosurgery (MCh and DNB)

In India, there are two types of training in neurosurgery. (1) A 3-year MCh program for those trainees who have undergone postgraduate training in general surgery (MS) and (2) a 6-year program for those who opt for neurosurgical training immediately after medical graduation. The qualification MCh (neurosurgery) degree is awarded by the universities or the institutes. The alternative is a national-level examination offered by the National Board of Examinations (India), leading to diplomat of national board qualification (DNB). The 6-year training program includes 1 year of training in general surgery and training in neurology, neuroradiology, neuropathology and neurosurgery. The trainees have to work on a research project and submit a dissertation or thesis at the time of final examination.

Royal Australasian College of Surgeons (RACS)

The training program training requirements include a successful completion of the RACS Fellowship Examination in Neurosurgery. The RACS Fellowship Examination in Neurosurgery is the final examination, at the standard and level of competency equivalent to that of a consultant surgeon in their first year of independent practice as a neurosurgeon. The examination comprises both a written and clinical/Viva component.

The RACS Fellowship Examination in Neurosurgery comprises both a written and clinical/Viva component. The clinical/Viva examination consists of five separate segments. At each Viva examination segment, the candidate is examined by a pair of examiners.

Clinical cases – 45 minutes

Candidates will be asked to examine and discuss several (usually three or four) patients in front of two examiners, with an emphasis on diagnosis and management of brain, spine and peripheral nerve conditions, as well as communication and patient interaction.

Neuroradiology – 25 minutes

Candidates will be shown 15–20 radiological images on a computer screen. They will be expected to demonstrate an understanding of the diagnosis and the clinical relevance of this diagnosis.

Surgical anatomy – 25 minutes

Candidates will be shown 15–20 computer images of relevant basic and applied anatomy. A level of knowledge is expected that demonstrates an understanding of the relationship between functional and structural anatomy.

Surgical pathology – 25 minutes

Candidates will be shown 15–20 computer images of pathological specimens, histological slides and correlative radiology. They will be asked to diagnose the pathology and relate this to the clinical outcomes and management.

Operative surgery – 25 minutes

Candidates will be shown three to four radiological images on a computer screen and asked to demonstrate knowledge of the operative approach to various neurosurgical conditions, including the management of intraoperative complications.

The results of the Examination will be declared at the conclusion of the examination.

Conclusion

There are essential differences in content and styles among the range of oral and clinical examinations across the world. Walking into the exam wherever you may be, having a very clear understanding of what the format entails is essential. Gaining as much information from websites of the examining bodies, attending preparatory courses and talking to recent candidates is the best way to avoid nasty surprises. Finding out at the last minute that you need to bring your own tendon hammer or that your attire does not meet with the expected dress code can give needless anxiety and seriously hamper your own chances of success.

If you are examined at a particular hospital, it may be useful to consider the expertise of that institution. Do they do a lot of functional work? Have they got a large paediatric unit? Are you likely to be examined by a particular examiner who has their own hobby horse subjects?

It is also worth spending some time on the logistics of the exam. If the exam is in another city make sure that travel plans leave plenty of time for possible delays. Ensure that the neighbourhood where you are staying is quiet and your hotel is as relaxing as possible. Have you worked out how long it takes to get from the hotel to the hospital? Are there decent places to eat? If you really need that caffeine shot is there somewhere to fuel up? These may seem like minor details, but the more preparation you do on these things the more you can set your mind to the exam itself.

There are two very important skills that are beneficial: **organization** and **examination skills**. There is a difference between a candidate who is well organized compared to a candidate who is randomly providing answers. Candidates with excellent examination skills will also have a clear advantage.

To improve your **knowledge**: read more with a critical eye; **skills**: practise and improve your weak areas; **confidence**: comes with knowledge, experience and practice.

Preparing for the neurosurgical examination is a challenge. Your revision must not be rushed. This book serves as a guide with which you can test yourself on examination-style questions and obtain the correct answers. This book covers all clinical sections of the examination in a comprehensive and structured manner. Organize your revision in a productive way in order to address the various conditions that will be encountered. This book serves as a guide and a revision aid, but it cannot replace examining patients with clinical signs in hospitals and outpatient settings. By acquiring the essential knowledge and skills and through independent study during your training, you will be able to communicate your knowledge to the examiners.

Assimilate your knowledge into clinical practise. Practise performing regular neurological examinations to ensure that you have a structured planned routine.

Enjoy the journey!

1 How to Succeed

Viva advice

Preparation for the oral and clinical neurosurgical exam should be well structured and organized. There are 'early' and 'late' phases. In the early phase, the emphasis is on acquiring knowledge. The sooner you begin the revision, not only will you be better prepared, the more relaxed you will be during the exam. One should minimize the risk by establishing what are the 'hot topics' – those that come up frequently, that have multiple areas to test the candidate and good tests of clinical reasoning. Our advice is to avoid extremes. On the one hand, you should not waste valuable time with in-depth research into highly specialized topics. On the other hand, avoid large gaps in your knowledge by only concentrating on the major topics. Ensure you have a clear revision timetable, a strategy to tackle the exam and a way to organize your notes and thoughts.

Allocation of time – Knowledge sampling

When it comes to the assimilation of knowledge, a simple fact remains – you cannot know absolutely everything. The key is to have insight into the 'high yield' topics (either written, knowledge-based, clinical technique or Viva discussion) and spend more time on these areas and less on those that are unlikely to be encountered. Developing a revision system to hone your knowledge is the key, especially when the examination dates loom close and increasing stress levels make these tasks more haphazard and less efficient.

For the neurosurgical exam, there is a core body of neurosurgical information that is essential, the **must know**. Beyond that there is additional knowledge and wisdom, which can be considered as **should know**, with a third sphere of content, which can be considered as **may know**. The examiner's task is to ensure that the exam candidate demonstrates a robust understanding of 'must know' topics to pass. Assessment of the 'should know' and 'may know' content is directed at determining the depth and breadth of neurosurgical training, which also serves as a surrogate marker to determine a 'rank' of sorts among peers. This strategy provides a structure with which to understand the selection of topics encountered within the oral and clinical exam.

Within the entire neurosurgical curriculum, there is, of course, a sub-division of topics. Taking the example of paediatric neurosurgery, the curriculum will encompass a number of topics, as illustrated in this 'knowledge cloud' (see Figure 1.1). Within this illustrative selection, the topics in the larger font will be generally considered 'must know', with the smaller fonts successively representing 'should know' and 'may know' domains. Considering the time limitations of the exams, the exam can only 'sample' a section of this knowledge cloud with Viva questions or clinical cases based on the topic chosen. The probability of an individual topic being selected for questioning

DOI: 10.1201/9781003254379-1

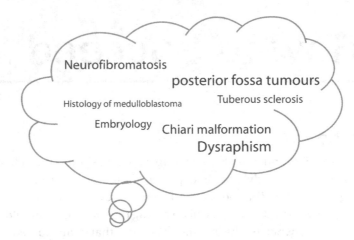

Neurofibromatosis

posterior fossa tumours

Histology of medulloblastoma   Tuberous sclerosis

Embryology   Chiari malformation

Dysraphism

Figure 1.1 Example of 'knowledge cloud' of paediatric neurosurgery topics.

is directly proportional to the importance of the topic as perceived by the examiner. Thus, the probability of 'must know' questions coming up is greater than 'should know' topics, which is greater than 'may know' questions.

These principles are commonly understood but often not considered either early on or very late in exam revision. When beginning the bulk of exam preparation, the key is to elucidate the 'probability algorithms' in the minds of the examiners, which are very well replicated if one were to *discuss the subspecialty with senior neurosurgeons* in your unit. For example, a paediatric neurosurgical consultant with several years' experience will be able to prioritize the 'must know/should know/may know' topics in paediatrics. This information is what needs to be understood to allocate exam preparation time to the topics, not the list of conditions listed in a neurosurgical exam preparation textbook.

With respect to the final stages of preparing for the exam, it is this prioritization that should determine the allocation of time needed to cover all topics. For example, on the evening before the exams, you should confirm that you have rehearsed your model answers on the key topics. It would be a better use of time to spend a few minutes perfecting the delivery of answers for such a topic rather than opening up a histopathology book to review the detailed findings of paraffin sections for a specific tumour. Though clearly the latter can be asked, an inability to answer the question will not fail a candidate. But a less polished, hesitant answer about the common differentials of brain tumours that requires prompting by the examiner can risk your performing below the accepted standard.

In essence, one needs to consider that only a small percentage of the entire curriculum is going to be sampled, and, by definition, one cannot know everything that can be asked. So it is important to bolster knowledge and delivery of answers for the more likely sampled topics rather than to devote equal time to all topics.

Late phase preparation

There is often a significant period of time between completion of the written component of the exam and commencement of the oral and clinical sections. This is an important 'late' phase of preparation. Factual knowledge has already been assessed in the written component, and the Viva is meant to explore your logical understanding of this assimilated information. *During this later stage of Viva revision, prepare the expected answer. There should be little new knowledge to acquire.* (Hence, the importance of the 'early' phase of preparation.) The experience of most candidates who have taken the oral and clinical components is that they overwhelmingly relied on their previous experience and knowledge rather than new information that they acquired during the 'late' phase of their preparation. Under stressful conditions, problem-solving skill defaults to past experience and pattern recognition. Managing performance during these stressful conditions is the key to success, and much can be gained by understanding how we perform within these scenarios, as detailed later.

There are numerous examples. During the operative Viva, there will be questions directed to how to avoid and address intra-operative complications, and, during the intermediate cases, what investigations are required to help obtain the underlying diagnosis. This strategy returns back to your preparation in the early phase. In addition to acquiring knowledge, you should be in the correct frame of mind in preparing for this exam in your daily practice. Take notes while on the wards, in the outpatient setting and in the operating room. We advise assembling a 'tool box' for examining patients. Some exams require you to take items with you to the exam. Your tool box will also provide helpful reminders on your order and the content of your neurological exam.

Assemble your 'tool box'

- Caliper.
- Coins of two denominations.
- Cotton wool balls.
- Key.
- Medical hat pins (red and white).
- Neurotips.
- Ophthalmoscope.
- Paper clip.
- Pen.
- Picture of a famous political figure (e.g. the Queen or the President of the United States).
- Ruler.
- Snellen's pocket eye chart.
- Tendon hammer (e.g. MDF Queen Square Hammer).
- Tongue depressor.
- Torch.
- Tuning forks (c128 Hz and c512 Hz).

Last-minute cramming is not rewarding. Finally, no matter how well prepared you are for the exam, it is challenging to answer a question that you have not prepared in advance. It is advised during your late preparation to select possible topics (surprisingly, these turn out to be fewer than you would have thought), imagine the various possible questions (putting yourself in the examiner's position) and prepare your final answers.

The skill of answering Viva questions

A very useful concept to understand performance in the exam is the Dreyfus model[1] of adult skill acquisition. After all, the exam is a platform to demonstrate your 'performance', and thus it can be vastly improved by studying the stepwise improvement inherent in any complex adult skill acquisition. The concept is perhaps best understood by considering the analogy of driving (see Table 1.1). The performance varies as tabulated from a novice who has to be told the exact rules of driving (when to exactly

Table 1.1 Dreyfus model of skill acquisition[1]

Level	Description	Analogy
Novice	• Rigid adherence to taught rules or plans • Little situational perception • No discretionary judgement	New learner driver who needs to be told the exact rules of driving, e.g. change gear from 1 to 2 when speed is greater than 10 mph, look at left and rear mirror when turning left, etc.
Advanced beginner	• Guidelines for action based on attributes or aspects (aspects are global characteristics of situations recognizable only after some prior experience) • Situational perception is still limited • All attributes and aspects are treated separately and given equal importance	With experience the 'advanced beginner' driver starts to notice the sound of the engine (high revs) as a cue to going up through the gears ... learns more cues or rules that determine driving, e.g. how close is the car in front (if too close need to go slower) and how close is the cyclist on the side, etc.
Competent	• Coping with crowdedness • Now sees actions at least partially in terms of longer-term goals • Conscious, deliberate planning • Standardized and routinized procedures	Driver starts to learn to 'ignore rules' as can't actively think about too many rules but starts to simply know intuitively how fast to go, which gear to take ... e.g. when late can start to make changes to drive faster, etc.
Proficient	• Sees situations holistically rather than in terms of aspects • Sees what is most important in a situation • Perceives deviations from the normal pattern • Decision-making less laboured • Uses maxims for guidance, whose meaning varies according to the situation	Driver goes into a turn with relatively high speed and just realizes that the car seems to be going too fast ... considers options of taking foot off accelerator pedals or breaking ... decides to gently depress break ... car achieves speed which driver is more comfortable with
Expert	• No longer relies on rules, guidelines or maxims • Intuitive grasp of situations based on deep tacit understanding • Analytic approaches are used only in novel situations when problems occur • Vision of what is possible	High-speed turn on wet road on motorway ... an 'expert' driver will intuitively take foot gently off accelerator to allow car to achieve and maintain the optimal speed ... all this can be happening while carrying on a conversation uninterrupted with passengers ... all actions are automatic

change gears, etc.) to an expert driver who can drive a car at high speeds at night in wet conditions without the passengers becoming uncomfortable on the turns.

Similarly, in a Viva exam situation, the ability to present can range from being a novice to an expert. The 'novice' will be thinking of the 'rules' of answering and trying to use them to formulate the answers. For example, when asked about a scan showing a left Sylvian fissure subarachnoid haemorrhage (SAH), the candidate will think, 'What is this? Is it a traumatic or spontaneous SAH? Should I use the WFNS or Fisher grade to describe it? What are the other things I should think of?'

An 'expert', on the other hand, may say, 'This 50-year-old female has a history typical of SAH and the scan confirms a Fisher grade 3, WFNS grade 1 spontaneous SAH with early hydrocephalus. I would bring the patient across urgently for a computed tomography angiogram (CTA) to investigate for a middle cerebral artery (MCA) aneurysm.'

The 'expert' is one who has become so experienced with dealing with a situation, presenting it before seniors and treating similar patients that the description of the scan and management plan comes automatically, and one does not have to think about what to say. It should be comforting to know that most candidates who attempt post-graduate exams will be at least at the 'competent' level or higher in dealing with most common cases. They therefore need to manage their stress levels to allow their level of 'skill acquisition' to shine through in the discussions they have with the examiners.

Managing stress

The Yerkes–Dodson law (Figure 1.2),[3] or the stress/performance curve, is a well-studied topic in various human endeavours. At its essence, this law merely states that initially performance improves with increasing levels of 'stress' or 'arousal'. However, beyond a certain point, further increases in stress result in worsening performance and are counterproductive. Though this principle was first scientifically demonstrated by Yerkes–Dodson in animal biological models over a century ago, it is

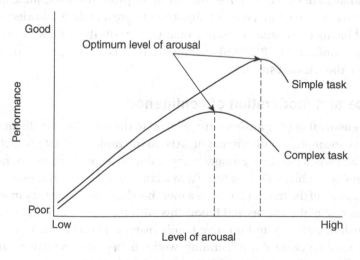

Figure 1.2 Yerkes–Dodson law.

grounded in common sense and has been shown to be appropriate for human biological responses as well.[4] What is important to realize is that the relationship between performance and stress is dependent on the complexity of the task being performed.

A natural corollary of this fact is that in a very stressful situation, such as a postgraduate exam, candidates will continue to perform well at a task that is 'easy' for them. (They will follow the curve to the right of the diagram.) During the same exam setting, they will invariably end up worse at tasks that are 'complex' for them (curve to the left). So if they were already 'proficient' (stage 4 of the Dreyfus model detailed earlier) at performing a fundoscopy examination, despite supra-normal stress levels, they may still continue to perform as if 'competent' at the examination and thus easily meet the criteria the examiners are looking for to pass a candidate. But a candidate who was 'competent' may drop down to the 'advanced beginner' stage and then find himself or herself in trouble in regard to meeting the minimum requirements expected.

It is therefore imperative that candidates do not alter or modify their examination techniques significantly close or on the day to the examination. Such changes to the subtle sequence of steps required to perform even a relatively simple task, without significant prior practice, will mean candidates will be more likely to behave as if the task is a 'complex' one, with a risk of poorer performance at high stress levels.

Performance in a post-graduate exam is just that – a performance. It involves a plethora of 'soft' skills, which complement the presentation of knowledge and application of the core medical subject being examined. These need to be presented at a 'competent' level or better and include the following:

- Verbal fluency;
- Syntax emphasis;
- Eye contact;
- Body language; and
- Confidence (a combination of the above).

Most candidates are concerned over the ability to present an adequate amount of content to the examiner, but it is more important to present their knowledge in a systematic and balanced approach and in a manner that fits the 'profile' that the examiner seeks to confirm. In FRCS(NS) examinations, this is the 'profile' of a first-day consultant in the relevant specialty.

Relevance and moderation of confidence

It is vital to ensure that your answers are relevant to the question. An illustration may be the classic example of a discussion of SAH. Many undergraduate books list mnemonics of the causes and interestingly many trainees seem to retain 'connective tissue disorders' (e.g. Ehlers–Danlos type IV, Marfan's syndrome and pseudoxanthoma elasticum) as one of the major causes. In a membership exam, one may inadvertently recite this as one of the causes and follow this with the more common causes, such as hypertension, smoking and positive family history. However, in a post-graduate exam, the examiner (who almost certainly would be a practising consultant) would not take kindly to such as starting with rare causes as the initial answer. The examiner

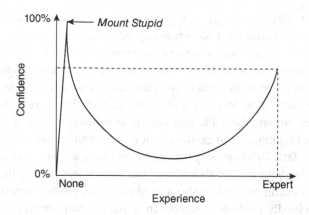

Figure 1.3 Dunning–Kruger effect (unskilled and unaware of it: how difficulties in recognizing one's own incompetence lead to inflated self-assessments). (From Kruger & Dunning, 1999.)

would be seeking to hear a clinically experienced discussion wherein the candidate may start by stating that the major risk factors are the most common pathologies. Further detailed discussions may end up with the probability of different pathologies causing SAH, its mechanism, treatment and recent publications on the subject. Key here is the chronology of the discussion, which represents the expected 'pattern' of behaviour and answers from a first-day consultant.

One should also think about the degree of confidence with which a reply is given. Of course, when answering a question on a subject that is expected to be a familiar part of general neurosurgical practice, e.g. management of extradural haemorrhage, it is entirely appropriate to display confidence in what you are talking about. If, however, the subject matter is one that even very experienced consultants find challenging, it is best to display an element of restraint even if you happen to be quite good at the particular operation. For example, a candidate launching headfirst into how they like to remove thalamic cavernomas with the impression that they do it every day, generally would not go down well. One might assume the candidate has so little experience that they do not realize that this is a challenging operation. This concept is illustrated by the Dunning–Kruger effect (Figure 1.3). If someone is speaking with great confidence, the choice the examiner has is either the candidate is really an expert or is very inexperienced and naive. In these exams, for complex procedures, the examiners would tend to assume that the candidate is in the naïve, inexperienced or maverick category. Ensure that your communication reflects that these pathologies can be difficult to treat and surgery is not without risks.

Taking advantage

Understanding the exam pattern and psychology of the examiners is the best aid a candidate can have for better performance. Knowing the basic facts is important. Usually, the Viva will start with simple topics, and then the questions will have a crescendo of increasing complexity. Therefore, it is not advised to start with a complex answer because this could be counterproductive; similarly, if you fail to adequately answer the remaining complex questions, this may not affect your overall score.

Provided it is not at the very beginning of the session, if you are asked about a topic that you are well prepared for, take advantage of this. You can guide the examiner through your answer to demonstrate your knowledge. The aim should be to obtain the 'gold medal' in these situations. Demonstrate that you are a safe neurosurgeon with a solid foundation in the basic topics. Most important, be attentive and listen to the examiners. They may provide hints and guide you in the correct direction. Most candidates underestimate the willingness of the examiners to help during the examination. With the vast majority of examiners, it is not a confrontation or an exercise in psychological warfare. This begins by the questions being asked and dictates how long and comprehensive your answer should be. The best strategy is to 'define, classify and then amplify'. For example, if asked about methods of evaluating cerebral blood flow (CBF), define, classify (invasive vs. non-invasive or quantitative vs. qualitative) and then amplify (mention the various investigations). However, if asked about the application of positron emission tomography (PET) scans in the estimation of CBF, concentrate on the details of this specific investigation. Similarly, during the clinical examination, if the examiner directs you towards examining a particular area, then take the hint and concentrate on this specific area to detect the abnormality. Moreover, the examiner will prompt you to move forward if you are taking too much time in irrelevant areas, or they may not interrupt you if the examination is relevant to diagnosing the underlying pathology. If the examiner repeats the question, it is likely that your answer is not appropriate.

Planning for specific scenarios

Throughout the oral and clinical neurosurgical examination, you will be provided with different scenarios for management. You must **listen** to the examiner and understand the question being asked. There are endless pitfalls. The following are important examples:

The examiner provided you with a long scenario on a polytrauma case. During the description, you are informed that the patient is localizing pain, making few incomprehensible sounds and not opening eye to pain. One pupil is noted to be fixed and dilated. It is best not to start your answer by reporting that you will first assess the patient's Glasgow Coma Scale (GCS) and pupils, as this information has already been provided. Similarly, if you are provided with a case in which the patient, a teacher, is suffering from intractable epilepsy despite medical optimization and is being considered for surgery, it is best not to report that you would optimize medical management in the first instance.

Once you have absorbed the information relayed in the question, you should take a moment to ask yourself 'what is the examiner REALLY asking?' Of course, there will be details specific to the particular scenario that the examiner will want to hear, but there will be an overall theme. Some examiners are testing whether you are a safe neurosurgeon. Are you going to talk about the various approaches to the pineal gland or actually get on and deal with the obstructive hydrocephalus for which has caused the acute deterioration? Do you have sufficient experience to predict common complications and ensure that you do everything to avoid them in the first place or if they should happen, know how to get yourself out of trouble? For example, craniotomy with an inter-hemispheric approach in the exam will potentially result in a breach of the superior sagittal sinus. Best to express all the measures you would take to avoid this complication in the first place, but if it does happen you should explain that you would need to warn the anaesthetist to watch his end-tidal CO_2 for air embolism, etc.

For some scenarios, there is no one right answer. They just want to kick you a ball and see where you go with it. They want to evaluate your thought process. Is it logical, sensible and achievable? In other cases, they are looking for one very specific piece of factual information instead of the endless list of options.

Understanding the purpose of the exam and the conduction of the assessment from the examiner's point of view as outlined in this book is useful. Essentially, demonstration of safety and applying knowledge to a specific case or situation are the main issues. The emphasis on safe practice is the key despite your excellent preparation and knowledge; failing the exam can happen when you lose concentration and when you give answers with detrimental outcomes. Examples of this include not addressing associated symptomatic hydrocephalus or performing a lumbar puncture or insertion of a lumbar drain, having forgotten that the presenting case has a significant intra-cranial mass lesion. Obviously, consistent demonstration of poor knowledge in several areas will result in a fail mark.

On the other hand, achieving excellence does not just depend on your standard or knowledge but also on the presentation of your answers within the allocated time for each question. The examiners are instructed to cover several topics within a given period of time. As such, their prompts are aimed to obtain the appropriate answer trying to help you rather than to intimidate you. During your preparation, the key is to predict common questions and topics that are favourable in exams. You should have in mind beforehand an average of three key points for each topic (usually demonstrating safety, complication avoidance and perhaps relevant anatomical nuances) that are prepared prior to your exam. Giving an answer that includes all these key points that are specifically relevant to the question without any prompting will achieve high marks.

Common pitfalls

There are four main reasons why candidates run into difficulties during the oral and clinical examination.

1 Not picking up on cues

Throughout the exam, the examiner will be providing you snippets of information. It is vital to LISTEN very carefully to what is being said and pick up on ways the examiner is trying to help you. An examiner having to repeat information because you didn't listen properly or worse still trying to shift your mindset back on track and being ignored will inevitably end in a fail. The exam is as much a test of listening as it is of speaking.

2 Poor presentation of answers

Although the topics and initial questions are standardized, the subsequent questions are based on your previous answers. With a degree of certainty, you can prepare for possible questions that will be asked on a given topic. Complex answers will generate subsequent difficult questions. If you do not know the answer, within reason, tell the examiner that you 'do not know' so you may move on to the next topic.

3 Lack of safe management

Before embarking on any complex management plan, it is important to demonstrate that you have considered all forms of treatment (e.g. conservative, medical and surgical). The term 'complication avoidance' requires pre-emptive knowledge of the potential complication and demonstration of the safeguards against these.

4 Misinterpretation of the evidence and non-malleable thinking

Ensure that you read the quoted literature from multiple sources. For example, stating that the International Subarachnoid Aneurysm Trial (ISAT) indicates that endovascular coiling is preferred to aneurysm clipping is correct. But in fact, the literature's findings relate to small (<10 mm) anterior circulation aneurysms. It is best to avoid the terms 'always' and 'never'. The examiner will set to prove you wrong. Moreover, this may represent non-malleable thinking. For example, the statement, 'I "always" use a lumbar drain in aneurysm surgery' will be followed by the examiner providing you with a scan of an MCA aneurysm with a large haematoma, contraindicating the role of a lumbar puncture. Similarly, providing exact figures or percentages should be avoided. This represents knowledge from limited sources.

References

1. Dreyfus S, Dreyfus H. *A five stage model of the mental activities involved in directed skill acquisition*. Berkeley, CA: Operations Research Center, University of Berkeley, 1980.
2. Eraut M. Non-formal learning and tacit knowledge in professional work. *Br J Educ Psychol* 2000; 70(1): 113–136.
3. Yerkes RM, Dodson JD. The relation of strength of stimulus to rapidity of habit-formation. *J Comp Neurol Psychol* 1908; 18: 459–482.
4. Sjöberg H. Interaction of task difficulty, activation, and workload. *J Human Stress* 1977; 3(1): 33–38.
5. Kruger J, Dunning D. Unskilled and unaware of it: how difficulties in recognizing one's own incompetence lead to inflated self-assessments. *J Pers Soc Psychol* 1999; 77(6): 1121–1134.

2 Clinical Intermediate and Short Cases

As a reminder, by the end of your history taking and prior to the start of the clinical examination, you should be aiming to have localized the pathological process, determined the underlying aetiology and established the indications and urgency for treatment. The actual clinical examination mainly serves to confirm your hypothesis. The majority of cases will be completed by looking at scans and discussing the management plans.

Remember to be economical with your time – if you have spent some time taking a history from a patient with an obvious expressive dysphasia when it comes to the examination instead of saying 'and now I would like to examine speech' start by saying 'I picked up several errors in speech on speaking to Mr X, including some paraphrasias and perseveration.' Or when you are asking the patient to walk to the examination couch, examine gait instead of doing it after they get off the examination couch.

For the current British FRCS (NS) examination, the two intermediate cases are of 20 minutes (7 minutes history, 7 minutes exam, 6 minutes investigations and management) and the four short cases are of 10 minutes each.

History taking

The intermediate cases

Taking a full history within the allocated time is essential. Your initial aim is to localize the lesion and to establish the pathological process. The subsequent history taking depends upon whether your given case is one that has not had definitive intervention vs. a case that has already been previously treated. Practicalities dictate that most patients appearing in these exams will have been already treated. Remember, however, that these cases are prone to last-minute changes and patients may be brought in from the ward at the last minute.

Box [1]: History-taking structure for the long cases with a pathological process (untreated and already treated)

Untreated
- Where is the lesion?
  - Look ++
  - Start focused examination
- What is the process?

DOI: 10.1201/9781003254379-2

- Should we operate?
- If so, how soon?

Already treated

- Where is the lesion?
  - Look ++ all scars
  - Start a focused examination
- What is the process?
- What is the impact of previous interventions on the patient?
  - Post-op complications
  - Epilepsy
  - RT
    - Cognitive function
    - Pituitary replacement
- Recurrence

The importance of localizing the lesion by taking a comprehensive history prior to conducting the physical examination cannot be overemphasized. Otherwise, a nontargeted examination may not only fail to establish the diagnosis but also will miss more subtle and relevant physical findings. As an example, if a patient describes difficulty with walking, then it is important to find out if it is because of the motor weakness of a particular movement, spasticity or impairment of balance. Then, take a history to localize the lesion within the neuroaxis if not due to nerve root or peripheral nerve origin. A spinal origin may have associated sensory manifestations in a dermatomal distribution or involve the upper limbs to indicate the approximate spinal level. Presentations associated with an intracranial origin include involvement somewhere along the motor pathways or the cerebellum in cases of gait ataxia. Seek the presence of telltale symptoms such as headaches or seizures. Appropriate cranial nerve deficits may indicate localization within the posterior fossa. This will direct your detailed neurological examination. The examination technique for eliciting motor deficit of spinal origin following a myotomal pattern differs from that of cerebral origin. Similarly, patients complaining of diplopia elicit a history focusing on such symptoms (e.g. facial numbness or bulbar and limb deficits), indicating whether the lesion is localized to the orbit, cavernous sinus or brainstem. Otherwise, when it comes to physical examination, you may miss a mild degree of proptosis or subtle sensory deficit in the V1 distribution.

Take the opportunity at this stage of history taking to pick up deficits even before you perform the actual examination. Examples include the pattern of dysarthria or speech deficits, involuntary movements such as tremors or hemifacial spasm, the presence of nearby walking sticks or hearing aids, posture and movements. If the patient mentions an external mass, skull defect or a traumatic scar and even a scar of some preliminary surgical procedure, being it a tracheostomy, a burr hole for biopsy or a shunt look at the exact site at this stage of the history taking as the location will dictate further relevant questions and guide your examination.

The history may indicate the underlying pathological process. It can be straightforward as in cases of trauma. The chronological duration of each symptom, the onset, course, progression and fluctuations may indicate a possible underlying aetiology. Although, in general, acute onset indicates a vascular insult, a progressive course may be associated with a neoplastic lesion. Be aware, a tumour may present acutely if a spontaneous intra-tumoural haemorrhage occurs. Repeated haemorrhages from a cavernoma can present with a fluctuating course.

Unless the patient is a poor historian or has cognitive dysfunction, if you are faced with a complex history that really cannot establish a reasonable localization or an underlying disease process, then think of syringomyelia, neurocutaneous syndromes (such as NF2 or Von Hippel–Lindau [VHL]) or other cases with multiple lesions (e.g. familial cavernomas). These are favourite cases to be selected for the clinical exams!

You will almost certainly be asked at the end of this session how would you manage this case. The indications for intervention almost entirely depend upon what you have established through your history taking. So do not terminate this part of the exam before establishing the severity of the current symptoms, neurological deficits and their specific impact on the patient's quality of life. The latter depends upon the patient's age, views, occupation and hobbies. Seeing a lesion on a scan without knowing whether it is incidental or symptomatic will cause dilemmas in dictating further management. Furthermore, the rate of progression of a particular symptom will dictate the speed and urgency of the required intervention. It is the extent and rate of deterioration rather than the size of the ventricles or of the tumour on imaging that indicates the urgency of CSF diversion or tumour resection.

When presented with a case that has already been treated previously during localization of the lesion, remember how useful it is to identify scars. If it can be done subtly, inquire during the history where scars are located. One has to be a little careful. Just jumping to asking a patient where their scars are before localizing the lesion clinically may well irritate the examiner. Also ensure that the patient declares all possible scars including those of possibly a previous EVD, ventriculostomy, shunt, tracheostomy or percutaneous gastrostomy. The location and configuration of the scar will dictate further questions regarding localization of the original pathological process. A localized retro-auricular scar indicates the possible location of the lesion in the CPA, while its partial extension inferiorly and anteriorly into the neck indicates that the lesion may be a glomus tumour or a jugular schwannoma with extracranial extension. With this information, you can direct your questions accordingly. Other scars will indicate the magnitude and possible lasting complications from previous treatment.

In such cases, beware that the purpose of selecting these cases perhaps was not merely for you to establish the original presentation, but rather there may be ongoing sequelae from previous interventions that necessitate assessment or recurrence that require re-intervention. Try to establish the impact of the original treatment on the quality of the patient's life. Events would include recurrent post-treatment shunt malfunction or post-operative adjuvant radiation therapy with resulting cognitive dysfunction or radiation-induced hypopituitarism requiring hormonal replacement. In fact, the purpose of the case may have been aimed for the candidate to assess post-operative epilepsy. Patients during the exam may not readily give this information regarding the impact of previous treatment unless asked. Especially, for neoplastic cases, find out the pattern of follow-up surveillance and establish whether or not recurrence occurred. In case of recurrence, establish if there were associated new symptoms or were merely detected on imaging as in that case, it will impact upon the proposed management plan.

Unless stopped by the examiner, you may try at the end of your history taking to directly ask the patient '*What investigations were carried out*?' '*What is planned for you regarding management*?' or '*What did they tell you regarding the options of treatment*?' This information will help you answering the final questions, but beware that what is provided may not really be the ideal answer!

The short cases

In the current FRCS exam, short cases do not have patients present and will often consist of photographs of clinical signs or investigations to work backwards to the clinical evaluation. This makes it easier for examiners to choose from a wider spectrum of cases. Previously, when the patient was present, it would be rare to be examined for neonatal disorders or a patient with a gunshot wound due to practical limitations. Now the examiners can be much more imaginative and cover larger portions of the neurosurgical syllabus.

Given the time constraints, one needs to be efficient in getting to the 'meat' of the case. The examiner will be pushing you on. Remember that the examiner is also under some stress. They have an obligation to get you through these cases in an allocated time. Listen carefully – in general, they are trying to assist you.

In your preparation, you should work through a wide selection of clinical signs. A lot of these are fairly predictable. Please prepare the predicted and subsequent questions that the examiner is likely to ask. For example, a common question is a photograph of a patient with a foot drop. There are several connotations of this. Is it due to a parasagittal meningioma? How would one differentiate from a peripheral nerve problem? If there are lower motor neurone signs? How does one differentiate a L4 or L5 radiculopathy vs. a common peroneal (e.g. external popliteal, lateral popliteal) palsy?

There are specific scenarios that are more or less approached in a standard fashion. Such examples include the facial features of acromegaly (also considered in cases of carpal tunnel syndrome) and Cushing's disease when the questions of a history of diabetes and hypertension should be asked.

Clinical examination

As previously explained, the examination starts when you take a history from the patient. Salient features (e.g. cognitive function, speech, posture, surgical scars, facial asymmetry, inattention and ophthalmoplegia) can be identified. Whilst taking the history, the localization of the pathological process should be achieved. This will enable you to perform a targeted neurological examination. Your clinical examination serves to confirm the diagnosis and determine the patient's overall management.

It is noteworthy that when you examine limb power it varies depending on whether it is targeted to assess intracranial or spinal function. For cranial cases, the general pattern of the motor weakness is global (e.g. evidence of a pronator drift). For spinal cases, inspect for specific muscle wasting and examine power in myotomal patterns. Avoid examining two movements sharing the same root or myotome value. It is recommended that you ask the patient to perform the movement to be examined and you oppose it rather than the other way round (e.g. for elbow extension, ask the patient to keep their arm straight and tell them to prevent you from flexing it). The reason is to examine a pure movement. If you ask them to straighten the elbow against resistance, there is a chance the patient may use 'trick' movements such as supination to compensate for a subtle extension weakness. As long as you demonstrate competence and identify the neurological deficit, the method you select will likely be acceptable. If the patient can walk or support their whole body weight on their tiptoes and heels, that will make the power in ankle movements MRC grade 5. Include the assessment of gait, Romberg's test and tandem walking (to assess the dorsal columns of the spinal cord).

During the intermediate and short cases, the candidate should have a systematic approach to obtaining a clinical history, performing the clinical examination, interpreting the appropriate investigations and obtaining the underlying diagnosis. A clear management plan should include conservative, medical and surgical treatments. Discussion regarding the patient's overall prognosis may also be included.

Remember to always be as courteous to the patient as possible. The examination is testing a candidate's interpersonal skills and their clinical acumen. This is how the examiner will evaluate how you treat patients on a daily basis. Being hurried or unthoughtful will create a poor impression. Inform the patient to ask you to stop if you are causing any discomfort or pain. An examiner will frequently tell you to skip certain unpleasant parts of the examination. Be prepared to stop a patient falling if you are performing Romberg's test or tandem walking; this can be achieved by standing behind the patient with an arm behind their back.

Having a balanced approach is important. A speedy, confident and thorough but targeted examination is recommended. Avoid a cursory and rapid examination because it will appear that you are going through the motions rather than actually examining the patient.

During your preparation, devise a logical and efficient scheme for the examination and be prepared to justify why you examine in a particular way. You will be assessed with the interpretation of the clinical signs and what further investigations are warranted. Formulate a list of possible cases and prepare your targeted answers.

The short cases

- Chiasmal/suprasellar lesions.
- Pituitary dysfunction.
  - Acromegaly.
  - Cushing's disease.
- Speech problems and assessments.
  - Dysphasia.
  - Dysarthria.
  - Dysphonia.

- Short history taking.
  - Facial pain, e.g. trigeminal neuralgia.
  - Headache, e.g. benign intracranial hypertension (BIH).
  - Seizure/syncope.
  - Transient neurologic deficit.
  - Hemifacial spasm.
- Cortical assessments, e.g. frontal, temporal, parietal and occipital lobes.
- Eyes.
  - Cranial nerve III palsy.
  - Diplopia.
  - Internuclear ophthalmoplegia (INO).
  - Carotico-cavernous fistula.
  - Parinaud's syndrome.
- Limbs.
  - Carpal tunnel syndrome.
  - Ulnar neuropathy.
  - Hemicord syndromes.
  - Brachial nerve palsy – ulnar, median and radial nerve palsies.
  - Myelopathy – cervical or thoracic.
  - Radiculopathy.
  - Numb hands/feet, e.g. peripheral neuropathy.
  - Foot drop.
- Gait.
  - Normal pressure hydrocephalus (NPH).
  - Cerebellar.
- Neurocutaneous syndrome.
  - Tuberous sclerosis.
  - Neurofibromatosis (NF-1, NF-2).
  - VHL syndrome.
  - Sturge–Weber syndrome.
  - Osler–Weber–Rendu syndrome.
- Functional.
  - Tremors.
  - Parkinson's disease.

Examples of the short cases

Cranial

- Assess this patient's speech.
- Assess this patient's swallowing.
- A patient presents with weakness in his right hand. Examine his frontal and parietal lobe function.
- A patient suffers from facial pain. Take a history and examine the patient.
- A patient suffers from gait imbalance. Perform the relevant examination.
- A patient suffers from headaches. Take a brief history and examine the patient.

Eyes

- A patient has blurred vision. Examine their eyes.
- A patient presents with ptosis, miosis and anhidrosis. Examine the patient for Horner's syndrome.
- A patient has a bulging eye. Assess for pulsatile proptosis.

Ears

- A patient suffers from tinnitus. Perform a focused neurological examination.

Endocrine

- A patient reports that he is no longer able to wear his wedding ring and his shoe size has increased. Perform the relevant examination.
- A patient reports weight gain despite careful dietary control. Perform the relevant examination.
- Spot diagnosis of acromegaly and Cushing's syndrome.

Functional

- A patient has a tremor. Perform a focused neurological examination.
- A patient suffers from long-standing seizures. Examine his temporal lobe function.
- A patient suffers from Parkinson's disease. Perform a focused examination.

Paediatrics

- Parents are concerned by their child's increased head size. Examine for craniosynostosis and classify the relevant subtypes.
- A child has been diagnosed with hydrocephalus secondary to a pineal tumour. Examine and investigate this child.

Spine

- A patient has a foot drop. Perform the relevant examination.
- A patient presents with reduced grip strength and dropping objects. Perform the relevant examination.

At the end, you may be asked the following:

- Summarize your findings.
- What is the likely diagnosis?

Define, classify and amplify

- Definition.
- Incidence.
- Aetiology.
- Causes: Use the mnemonic: INVITED MD.
  - **Infection.**
  - **Neoplasia.**

- Vascular.
- Inflammatory/immune.
- Trauma.
- Endocrine.
- Degenerative.
- Metabolic.
- Drugs.
- Pathophysiology.
- Clinical presentation.

- What would you do next?
- How would you manage this patient?
- What treatment options are available for this patient?
  - Conservative.
  - Medical.
  - Radiological.
  - Surgical.
- What is the overall prognosis?

Illustrative short cases

Case 1

You are asked to examine this patient.

Q1: Please examine and describe the salient features of this patient.
Stand at the end of the patient's bed.

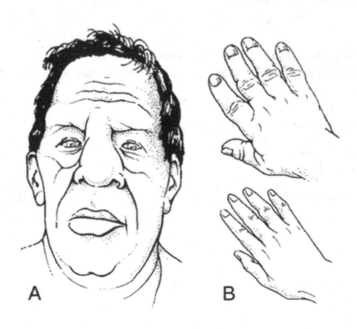

- **Inspection**: Look at the face.
  - Describe the coarse facial features – frontal bossing, large nose, prognathism.
  - Ask patient to open mouth, stick tongue out (large tongue) and to say 'arghh'. Coarse voice may be noted.
  - Examine hearing (e.g. conductive hearing loss).
- Ask to examine the hands.
  - Large and sweaty fingers.
  - Perform Tinel and Phalen's tests.
  - Examine the ulnar nerve.
- At the end of the examination, you may say to the examiner: 'To complete the examination I would review the patient's blood pressure and pulse, assess the patient's visual fields and perform a urine dipstick test to check for glucose.'

Spot diagnosis: Acromegaly

Case 2

Q1: *Please examine this patient's hands.*

Inspection

- Place both hands on the patient's lap or on a pillow.
- Compare both hands – dorsal and palmar aspects.
- Describe the wasting and weakness of the small muscles of the hand and partial clawing of the ring and little finger.
  - Comments – wasting of the first dorsal interosseous muscle.
  - The little finger may be abducted – Wartenberg's sign.
  - Finger clubbing (e.g. sign of Pancoast's tumour of the lung).
  - Petechial haemorrhages (e.g. vascular compromise – thoracic outlet syndrome).

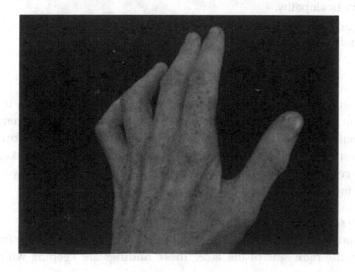

Normal   **Froment's positive**

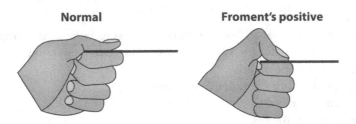

- Ask the patient to lift arms and then inspect medial epicondyle.
- Examine supracondylar region.
- Perform Tinel's test at the elbow.

Power

- Dorsal interossei abducts the index, middle and ring fingers.
- Adductor digiti minimi abducts the little finger.
- Adductor pollicis adducts the thumb (e.g. Froment's sign).
- Flexor digitorum profundus flexes the wrist, metacarpophalangeal and interphalangeal joints.
- Flexor carpi ulnaris flexes and adducts the wrist joint.

Sensation

- Light touch and pinprick – assess medial 1½ fingers.

Differential diagnosis

- Ulnar nerve palsy.
- Brachial neuritis.
- Pancoast's syndrome.
- Thoracic outlet syndrome.
- Cervical radiculopathy.

Spot diagnosis: Ulnar nerve palsy

Case 3

You have been referred a patient diagnosed with trigeminal neuralgia by a GP for consideration of surgical intervention. He has not responded to carbamazepine. He has severe pain in the right V1 distribution. He says that cold air and brushing his teeth does not bother him, but the pain can be triggered by alcohol intake. He tends to get a very runny nose when it comes on. It comes in spells. He shows you a photograph of his face during an episode.

What can be seen in the photograph?
The gentleman has right miosis and partial ptosis. I would also assess for reduced sweating on the right side of the face. These findings are keeping with Horner's syndrome.

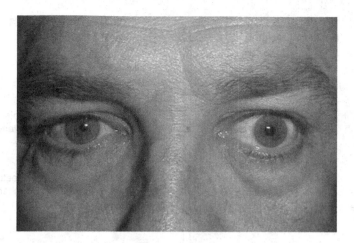

Explain the orders of neurones involved in sympathetic supply to the eye and give an example of a disorder that can affect each?

- **First order**. Hypothalamus to spinal cord – lateral medullary syndrome (Wallenberg syndrome).
- **Second order**. Ciliospinal centre of Budge via C8, T1, T2 to the superior cervical ganglion – Pancoast tumour.
- **Third order**. Superior cervical ganglion, carotid sheath, longus coli, CN VI, CN V1, to Muller's muscles – post-ACDF.

Do you think the GP was correct to diagnosis trigeminal neuralgia and would you recommend surgical intervention?

No. I suspect the gentleman has cluster headache and I would refer on my neurology colleagues for medical management.

Case 4

A nine-month-old child is brought in by his parents with concern about the flattening of the back of his head. Please examine.

Inspection

- Look for signs of syndromic features, including hypertelorism, midface deformities and limb deformities.
- Inspect for evidence of irritability, failure to thrive, macrocephaly, fullness of anterior fontanelle and for sun setting, which raise suspicion of increased intercranial pressure (ICP).
- Inspect from top the head shape – in positional plagiocephaly, the ipsilateral ear and forehead are pushed forwards and the contralateral ear and occiput backwards (parallelogram). In lambdoid synostosis, the ipsilateral ear is deviated posteriorly and the contralateral forehead and occiput show compensatory growth (trapezoid).
- Inspect from top the head shape – in positional plagiocephaly, the ears are level in height. In synostosis, the involved ear is deviated inferiorly and there

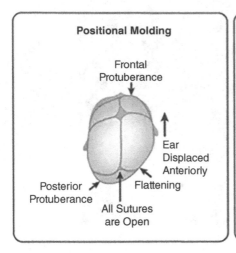
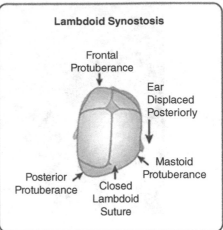

is a mastoid protuberance alongside a contralateral compensatory parietal contralateral bulge.

Palpation
- Palpate sutures.
- Palpate anterior fontanelle.

Other
- Cranial index measurement.
- Check eye movements, offer fundoscopy.

Are further investigations required?
In the case of positional plagiocephaly, the diagnosis is generally made clinically with appropriate reassurance of the parents. When there is concern about craniosynostosis, one should consider:

- Clinical photography.
- CT head scan.
- Genetic assessment.

Would you consider ICP monitoring?
It is an option if there are clinical features suggestive of raised intracranial pressure, but this needs to be addressed by a specialized craniosynostosis team.

Illustrative Intermediate cases

Common cases
- Pituitary tumours or sellar pathology.
  - Cushing's disease.
  - Acromegaly.
  - Craniopharyngiomas.

- Cerebellopontine angle tumours.
  - Acoustic neuroma.
  - Neurofibromatosis type 2.
  - Glomus jugulare tumours.
- Low-grade glioma.
- Radiation-induced meningioma.
- Cranio-cervical pathology.
- Syringomyelia.
- Chiari malformation.
- Meningioma.
- Spinal pathology.
- VHL syndrome.
- Brainstem cavernoma.
- Vascular.
  - Aneurysms.
  - Arteriovenous malformations (AVMs).
  - Carotid cavernous fistula (CCF).
- BIH.
- NPH.

History taking

Preparation

Ensure you take a targeted history in the allocated time allowed.

Introduce yourself to the patient.

Ensure adequate privacy.

You may ask the examiner to serve as your chaperone.

Targeted history taking

Obtain the patient's name, age, handedness and occupation.

Establish the presenting complaint (PC).

Obtain the history of the presenting complaint (HPC).

- Chronological order of the symptoms: time course, onset, duration, frequency, progression, location, quality, quantity, severity, aggravating and relieving factors and associated symptoms.
- Risk factors for the presenting complaint.
- System-specific questions related to presenting complaint.
- Investigations and treatment provided to date.

Past medical/past surgical/past anaesthetic history (PMH/PSH/PAH)

- **Use the mnemonic**: THREADS MIJ.
  - Tuberculosis.

- **H**ypertension.
- **R**heumatic fever/Rheumatoid arthritis.
- **E**pilepsy.
- **A**sthma.
- **D**iabetes.
- **S**troke.
- **M**yocardial Infarction.
- **J**aundice.

Medication and known allergies

Note all medications that the patient is taking and any known allergies.

Family history (FH)

First-degree relatives with relevant familial diseases.

Social history (SH)

- Marital status.
- Occupation.
- Smoking habit (number of pack-years).
- Alcohol intake (units/week).
- Exposure to industrial toxins.
- Recreational drug use.
- Living accommodation.
- Level of support (family and carers).
- Hobbies.

Review of systems

During your targeted history taking, ask only the relevant questions based on the patient's history.

Cardiovascular system

Chest pain, dyspnoea, orthopnoea, palpitations, dizziness, ankle swelling.

Respiratory system

Dyspnoea, exercise tolerance, paroxysmal noctural dyspnoea, wheeze, chest pain, cough, haemoptysis, hoarseness, fever.

Gastrointestinal system

Change in appetite, diet regimen, weight loss (amount and duration), dysphasia, odynophagia, regurgitation of foods/liquids, indigestion, nausea, vomiting, haematemesis, abdominal pain, abdominal distention, change in bowel habit, rectal bleeding, flatulence, jaundice.

Urogenital system

Abdominal pain, frequency of micturition, dysuria, urgency, polyuria, colour of urine, haematuria, nocturia, impotence, sensation of incomplete voiding.

Central and peripheral nervous system

Fits, faints or funny turns, headache, loss of consciousness, tremor, muscle weakness, paralysis, sensory disturbances, paraesthesia, sphincter dysfunction, alteration in senses (e.g. vision, hearing, touch, smell and taste), change in behaviour or personality.

Musculoskeletal system

Muscle, bone or joint pain, deformity, swelling, stiffness, limb weakness, decreased range of movement, functional loss.

Metabolic system

Change in weight and appetite, alteration of build and appearance.

Summary

Use key words to describe the salient features.

Clinical examination

1. Introduction and consent

- Wash/gel your hands.
- Introduce yourself to the patient and ask permission to examine them.
- Ensure adequate exposure of the patient.
- Check the patient's surroundings (e.g. walking or hearing aids, oxygen, drains, catheters, dressings).
- Inspect the patient as a whole (e.g. well – unwell/cachectic – obese/in pain – comfortable) including peripheral stigmata of underlying neurological disease, involuntary movements, abnormal facial expression.

2. Mental state evaluation

- **Appearance and behaviour**
  Does the patient appear self-neglected, depressed or anxious; do they behave appropriately; have they experienced mood changes; are they appropriately concerned about their symptoms?
- **Mood**
  Describe their current mood.
- **Systematic symptoms**
  Is there a history of weight loss or gain, sleep disturbance, appetite changes, constipation, changes in libido or anxiety?

- **Delusion, hallucination and illusion**

  Delusion: A firmly held belief, not altered by rational argument and not based on conventional belief within a culture or society.

  Hallucination: A perception experienced without external stimuli that is indistinguishable from the perception of a real external stimulus.

  Illusion: A misinterpretation of an external stimulus.

3. Higher function evaluation

- **Attention and orientation**
  - **Attention**. Digital span: Ask the patient to repeat a set of numbers (e.g. telephone number).
  - **Orientation**. Mini Mental State Examination (time, place, person).
- **Memory**.
  - **Immediate recall and attention**. Name and address. Ask the patient to remember a specific name and address and ask the patient to immediately repeat it back to you.
  - **Short-term memory**. After 5 minutes, ask the patient to recall the name and address.
  - **Long-term memory**. Ask the patient to name the President of the United States or Prime Minister.
- **Calculation**.
  - **Serial sevens**. Ask the patient to take 7 from 100, then 7 from 93 and so on.
- **Abstract thought (frontal lobe function)**.
  - **Proverb**. Ask the patient to explain a proverb: 'A stitch in times saves nine.' 'A rolling stone gathers no moss'.
- **Spatial perception (parietal and occipital lobe function)**.
  - **Clock face**. Ask the patient to draw a clock face and fill in the numbers. Then ask the patient to draw in the hands for the time 12:30 pm.
  - **Five-pointed star**. Ask the patient to copy a five-pointed star.
- **Visual and body sensory** perception **(parietal and occipital function)**.
  - **Recognize famous faces**. Show the patient a picture of the President of the United States, the Prime Minister or the Queen.
  - **Body perception**. Ask the patient to show the index finger and ring finger.
  - **Left and right perception**. Ask the patient to touch the right ear with the left index finger. Cross your hands and ask the patient which is your right hand.
  - **Sensory perception**. Ask the patient to close the eyes. Write a number or letter on their hand and ask the patient to report the number or letter (Agraphatesia-impaired ability to recognize letters or numbers drawn by an examiner's fingertip on the patient's skin.)
- **Apraxia.**
  - **Object recognition**. Ask the patient to close their eyes. Place an object (e.g. coin, key, paper clip) in the patient's hand and ask them to identify the object.

Three-hand test. Ask the patient to copy your hand movements. (Astereognosis is the inability to identify objects by feel only, in the absence of input from the visual system).

1. Make a fist and tap it on the table with your thumb facing upward.
2. Straighten out your fingers and tap on the table with your thumb facing upward.
3. Place your palm flat on the table. (Agnosia is the inability to interpret sensations and hence to recognize things, typically as a result of brain damage.)

4 Language evaluation

To evaluate for dysphasia, first establish that there is no higher mental dysfunction or a confusional state. Exclude other speech disorders (e.g. dysarthria and dysphonia). To simplify, the different types of dysphasia are *expressive, receptive, conductive* and *dysnomial*. Expressive dysphasia is localized in the dominant posterior inferior frontal gyrus and frontal operculum (Broca's area). Receptive dysphasia is localized to the dominant posterior superior temporal gyrus and the inferior parietal lobule (Wernicke's area). Conductive dysphasia results from white matter tract disruption, located in the arcuate fasciculus. (Other tracts are being investigated.) It is worth noting that in a large number of post-operative cases, conductive dysphasia is common and likely to be assessed in this examination. Dysnomial dysphasia (inability to recall words or names) is not well localized. It may involve a breakdown in one or more pathways in different areas of the brain, including the parietal and temporal lobes.

The clinical evaluation of speech should be performed in quick and clear successive steps.

Provide the examiner with a concluding statement at the end of each step.

Step 1: Ask the patient a question that requires a long and multi-sentenced answer.

Unless there is profound dysphasia, this step will assess higher mental function and orientation. It will be clear if the patient is suffering from an expressive dysphasia. Questions that are answered by short responses could potentially cause one to miss important speech deficits. For example, asking the patient to name various objects or colours is not sufficient.

Step 2: Determine whether the patient comprehends a complex task or discussion.

Do not rely on asking the patient to obey simple tasks because you may miss a receptive dysphasia.

Step 3: Ask the patient to repeat a long sentence.

Repetition assesses for a conductive dysphasia, which is characterized by intact auditory comprehension, fluent speech production and poor speech repetition.

Step 4: Ask the patient to name certain objects.

Naming assesses for dysnomial dysphasia. The patient will have problems recalling words and names.

Step 5: Ask the patient to read a section of a newspaper or book.

Reading assesses for dyslexia. The patient will have an impaired ability to recognize and comprehend the written word. They may have difficulty in reading fluently, despite normal or above normal intelligence.

Step 6: Ask the patient to write a few sentences.

Writing assesses for dysgraphia. The patient will have difficulty writing (handwriting and possibly coherence).

Assessment of speech is regarded as a simple concept as actually the correct approach is evaluation of the complex language function. Especially, when evaluating cases such as low-grade gliomas involving the language pathways, awareness of existence of the ventral and dorsal streams and phonemic and semantic paraphasias.

Dysphasia

Receptive

Start with simple questions. Ask the patient to report their name, date and location.

Ask the patient to obey simple commands, such as close your eyes (visual command).

Expressive

Ask the patient to name objects, for instance, to describe what they eat for breakfast.

Repetition

Ask the patient to repeat 'no ifs, ands or buts' and 'the sun is shining'.

Reading

Ask the patient to read a sentence.

Writing

Ask the patient to write a simple sentence.

Dysarthria

Ask the patient to repeat: 'British constitution', 'West Register Street' and 'Baby hippopotamus'.

Dysphonia

Ask the patient to cough and to say a sustained 'eeeeee'. Is there evidence of fatigue?

Listen to the patient's pitch, quality and tone of voice.

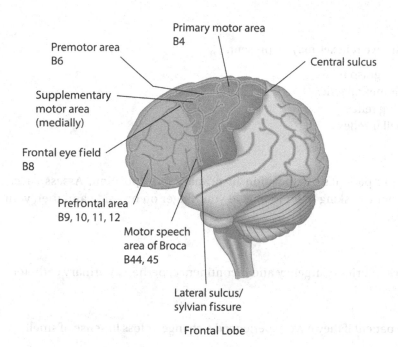

Primary motor area
B4

Premotor area
B6

Central sulcus

Supplementary
motor area
(medially)

Frontal eye field
B8

Prefrontal area
B9, 10, 11, 12

Motor speech
area of Broca
B44, 45

Lateral sulcus/
sylvian fissure

Frontal Lobe

5 Lobe evaluation

Lobe evaluation is an essential component of the neurological examination.

a. Frontal lobe.
b. Parietal lobe.
c. Temporal lobe.
d. Occipital lobe.

a Frontal lobe

Attention and orientation

Attention. Digital span: Ask the patient to repeat a set of numbers (e.g. telephone number).

Orientation. Mini Mental State Examination (e.g. time, place and person).

Behaviour

Assess for apathy or disinhibition.

Motor

Look at the patient's posture and gait. Do they have the typical flexed upper limb and extended lower limb of spastic hemiparesis (pyramidal weakness) and circumducting gait? Test for pronator drift. You can do traditional motor examination of the upper and lower limbs but be mindful that you are not looking for weakness in a nerve root or peripheral nerve distribution with a brain lesion.

Speech

Broca's dysphasia (pars triangularis and pars opercularis of the inferior frontal gyrus): Damage to this area results in expressive asphasia. Ask the patient to repeat: 'baby hippopotamus'.

Primitive reflexes

The primitive reflexes may be present.

- Palmar grasp reflex.
- Palmomental reflex.
- Rooting reflex.
- Glabellar reflex.

Frontal eye fields

Assess the patient's eye position in primary gaze position. Assess saccadic eye movement by asking them to look at your finger on one side and then your fist on the other.

Bladder function

Evidence of urinary urgency and incontinence, perhaps a urinary catheter.

Sense of smell

Ask the patient if they have experienced a change or loss in sense of smell.

Gait

Assess for a 'magnetic' gait.

Luria's test: This is a test of executive dysfunction. You make a fist, then put your hand down on its side, then flat (fist-edge-palm) and ask the patient to copy it. The patient may struggle because of difficulties with sequencing, working memory, planning and perseveration.

Abstract thought

Ask the patient to interpret 'A stich in time saves nine' or 'A rolling stone gathers no moss'.

Other neuropsychology tests

- Lexical fluency – generate as many words beginning with a letter
- Conceptualization – in what way are a banana and an orange alike?
- Working memory – recall a telephone number.

b Parietal lobe

Establish the patient's dominant hand. This will enable the candidate to use the appropriate neurological examination for the affected area.

General function of parietal lobes (e.g. applicable to both hemispheres).

Cortical sensory function

- **Sensory perception**
  - Ask the patient to close their eyes. Write a number or letter on the patient's hand and ask them to report the number or letter (e.g. graphaesthesia).

- **Tactile location/two-point discrimination**
    - Ask the patient to close their eyes. Touch a certain point on the patient's skin surface. Then ask the patient to indicate the location of the previously touched point. The expected accuracy is a few millimetres on a fingertip and may be even 5–10 cm on the back.
    - Ask the patient to close their eyes. Use a caliper or a fashioned paper clip to touch one or two points. Ask the patient if they feel 'one' or 'two' points.
- **Stereognosis**
    - Ask the patient to close their eyes. Ask the patient to identify objects (e.g. coin and key) in each hand (**astereognosia** – inability to perform this action).
- **Tactile extinction (sensory inattention)**
    - Test individual body parts on opposite sides of the body and simultaneously. Ask the patient to close their eyes, then touch the patient on both sides of the body, simultaneously initially and then alternately. Ask the patient to tell you when you are touching them (e.g. right hand; both hands; and left face and right hand). To make the test more sensitive, test different body parts at the same time (e.g. face and hand).
    - Patient ignores or denies any neurological deficit on the affected contralateral side of the body (hemi-asomatognosia, sensory neglect).

Visual fields

Assess for an inferior quadrantanopia.

Activities of daily living (ideomotor apraxia)

Ask the patient to comb their hair, drink a cup of tea or button their shirt/jacket.

Specific function of the parietal lobe (depending on hemispheric dominance)

1. In the dominant hemisphere

Gerstmann's syndrome – Dominant parietal lobe

Left-right dissociation	Cross your hands and ask the patient which hand is right and left.
Acalculia	Patient is unable to perform calculations – serial 7s.
Agraphia	Patient is unable to write.
Finger agnosia	Patient is unable to distinguish fingers [left index from the left thumb].

Left-right disorientation

Ask patient to touch their right ear with their left thumb.

Calculation

Serial sevens

Ask the patient to take 7 from 100, then 7 from 93, and so on.

Finger agnosia

Ask the patient to show the index finger and ring finger. Ask the patient to name fingers (finger agnosia).

Dyspraxia (ideo, ideomotor and motor)

2. In the nondominant hemisphere

Spatial perception (parietal and occipital lobe function)

- **Clock face**. Ask the patient to draw a clock face and fill in the numbers. Then ask the patient to draw in the hands for the time: e.g. 12:30 pm.
- **Five-pointed star**. Ask the patient to copy a five-pointed star (constructional apraxia).

Geographical dyspraxia

- The patient is unable to locate defined places or known locations.

Dressing apraxia

- Ask the patient to put on an inside-out jumper.

c *Temporal lobe*

Memory

Assess for impaired immediate recall and attention. Name and address: Ask the patient to remember a name and address and ask the patient to immediately repeat it back to you.

Assess for impaired short-term memory. After 5 minutes, ask the patient to recall the name and address.

Assess for impaired long-term memory. Name the President of the United States or the Prime Minister.

Speech

Wernicke's dysphasia (posterior part of the superior temporal gyrus): Damage to this area results in a receptive aphasia. The patient is unable to understand what has been said, e.g. unable to execute commands. Ask the patient to follow a command: 'When I clap my hands, and not before, touch your left ear with your right hand'. Note that the command must be delivered with no nonverbal communication. Also, beware of concurrent hemiplegia impairing the test.

Hearing

The primary auditory cortex lies in the temporal lobe (Heschl's gyrus). Although worth mentioning in the exam, it is very hard to assess clinically given that hearing is represented bilaterally.

Visual fields

Visual field (the optic radiation or geniculo-calcarine tract) defects result from damage to Meyer's loop resulting a superior quadrantanopia ('pie in the sky') and loss of colour vision.

Recognition of faces (prosopagnosia)

- Ask the patient to identify pictures of the President of the United States, the Prime Minister or the Queen.

d Occipital lobe

Visual fields

- If one occipital lobe is damaged, this can result in a homonymous hemianopsia.
- Occipital lesions may also cause visual hallucinations.
- Lesions in the parietal–temporal–occipital association area are associated with colour agnosia, movement agnosia and agraphia.

Illustrative cases

Case 1 (Frontal lobe examination)

A 64-year-old woman presents with a 5-year history of personality change and is now admitted with a generalized seizure (Figure 2.1).

Q1: What is the likely diagnosis?

This MRI scan demonstrates a large well-defined mass with mild surrounding oedema in the interhemispheric fissure of the frontal lobe. These features are suggestive of an olfactory groove meningioma.

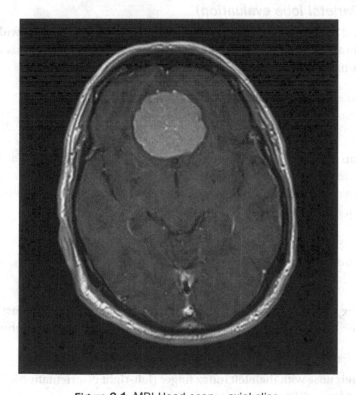

Figure 2.1 MRI Head scan – axial slice.

Q2: With this in mind, demonstrate the relevant positive neurological signs.
Because the MRI scan demonstrates a medial frontal lobe lesion, it is appropriate to proceed with a general examination followed by a focussed evaluation of the frontal lobe and cranial nerves (including the olfactory and optic nerves).

Inspection

- Appearance and behaviour.
- Comments about the position of the patient's eyes.
- Assess for saccadic eye movement (frontal eye fields).

Ask the patient a few brief questions

- MMS (time, place, person).
- Interpret 'A rolling stone gathers no moss' (abstract thinking).
- Ask about the sense of smell.
- Ask about bladder function.

Ask the patient to raise their arms

- Comments about pronator drift or motor weakness.
- Elicit grasp reflex.
- Pout reflex.
- Palmomental reflex.

Assess the patient's gait and mobility

Look for difficulty initiating movement, magnetic gait, short strides, difficulty turning.

Case 2 (Parietal lobe evaluation)

A 58 year old experienced mathematics teacher has recent problems with reduced concentration and intermittent headaches. There are disruptions in his classroom during lessons. An head MRI scan is arranged (Figure 2.2).

Q1: Perform a focussed, relevant examination for this patient.
Introduce yourself and ask permission to examine the patient.

Inspection

Comment on general appearances. Look for a scar (the scan shows what appears to be a burr hole overlying the lesion). The lesion looks like a Glioblastoma Multiforme (GBM), but a metastasis is a possibility and therefore there could be systemic features of neoplasia.

Ask the patient a few brief questions

- Hand dominance.

Assess the patient's speech

One might expect more receptive problems, and it is important to demonstrate this to the examiner. If there is time, a full assessment of language would be recommended.

Ask the patient to follow the following instructions (Gerstmann syndrome)

- Touch their nose with their left index finger (left-right disorientation).
- Name the fingers (finger agnosia).

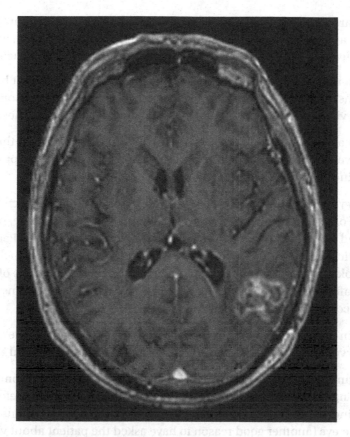

Figure 2.2 MRI Head scan – axial slice.

- Ask the patient to perform simple mathematics – serial sevens (dyscalculia).
- Test writing (agraphia).

Ask the patient to show their hands

- Pretend to write number on the palm of the hand (agraphastesia).
- Place coin in palm (astereognosia).
- Test for sensation/neglect (sensory inattention).
- Two-point discrimination.

Assess the patient's visual fields

Whilst you are testing, predict which quadrant is likely to be involved and spend extra time assessing that quadrant.

Q2: *What is the reason for the disruption in his classroom?*
This may be attributed to a combination of dysphasia and dyscalculia.

6 Detailed cranial nerve (I–XII) evaluation

Examination of the cranial nerves may seem like a familiar part of clinical evaluation, but it is interesting how easily candidates can be thrown off when an examiner asks 'please examine the face' (i.e. V and VII) or 'please examine the eyes' (i.e. II, III, IV, VI) instead of the specific cranial nerves. The cranial nerves extend over a large anatomical area, and one will often have to think 'which cranial nerves are important here?' In a patient with a history highly suggestive of a CP angle lesion, a candidate may be challenged why they are starting with the examination of the smell and eyes.

Smell: Often all that is required is a short question asking if the patient has noticed any problems with their smell. It may well be that the examination room does not have testing vials or 'sniffin sticks', but if they are available, please use them.

Eyes: When asked to examine the eyes begin by asking the patient if they can see with both eyes. If the patient is blind in one eye, then it would be inappropriate to cover the blind eye when examining the visual fields.

Inspect the eyes. Remember, there may be more signs in addition to cranial nerve pathology. For example, the patient may have proptosis. In such a case, one should stand behind the seated patient to examine the degree of proptosis. Perhaps they have a caroticocavernous fistula, and there is a helpful stethoscope dangling beside the bed. Look out for ptosis, and if present, remember the three orders of neurones that can be affected. Also, inspect their glasses. There may well be prisms inserted if someone is complaining of diplopia.

The two main components of this examination are the assessment of the optic nerve (**cranial nerve II**) and of the eye movements (**cranial nerves III, IV and VI**).

Start by examining the direct and consensual light reflex and accommodation. Perform swinging light test to assess for a relative afferent pupillary defect (RAPD) only if it is indicated. This defect is more likely to be present in patients with poor vision in one eye (another good reason to have asked the patient about vision prior to the start of this examination). The one pitfall includes bringing the light torch into the patient's field of view while shining the light because the pupillary reaction could result in accommodation rather than assessing the light reflex.

When assessing visual acuity, ensure that the patient is at the correct distance from the Snellen chart. In addition, you should not hold the reading chart, such as the Jaeger chart, but rather let the patient hold it at their own reading distance.

To examine visual fields by confrontation, ensure that the hat pin is equidistant between yourself and the patient. Assess for an enlarged blind spot. There is debate on whether the hat pin should be red or white. A loss of red colour vision occurs early in lesions of the optic nerve and optic chiasm. A red hat pin is a sensitive way to detect defects as a result of pathological processes in this region of the pituitary and suprasellar fossa. When you are examining for a retrochiasmatic lesion (e.g. homonymous hemianopia), the red colour becomes irrelevant. You may well already have had a strong clue about the location of the lesion – perhaps you have already gone so far as to say you think the lesion is in the left parietal lobe. Therefore, before starting the neurological examination start thinking, 'where is the field defect likely to be?' If it is a left parietal lesion one would expect a right inferior quadrantanopia.

During this part of the examination, there can be major challenges. The visual fields of both eyes overlap; therefore, each eye is tested independently. The patient should cover the right eye with the right hand (vice versa when testing the opposite eye). Use a red hat pin as the moving target. Start outside the usual 180° visual field, then move slowly to a more central position until the patient confirms visualization of the target. All four quadrants (upper and lower, temporal and nasal) should be tested. If the object is nearer to the patient than to you, you will detect a visual field defect that does not exist. If one has time, it is nice to map out the patient's blind spot, especially if there is a possibility of papilloedema or optic atrophy.

While examining the eyes, if you detect a visual field defect, it is important to examine cranial nerves III, IV and VI. In cases of pituitary macroadenoma invading the cavernous sinus, these cranial nerves may all be involved. If the question was specifically to examine the eye movements, then take your time to complete this task. Similarly, during fundoscopy, if the examiner does not report that the fundi are normal and prompts you to move forward, take your time to inspect both fundi because an abnormality may be present.

When examining eye movements, include the assessment of pursuit and saccadic movements and the presence of nystagmus. Ask the patient to report diplopia (double vision) because failure to talk to the patient during the examination may lead to an incomplete illustration of the underlying deficit. If there is evidence of uncoordinated movements without diplopia, ask the patient if they have been diagnosed with a squint. In patients with diplopia, cover alternate eyes to establish which suppresses the false image. This is important to differentiate between subtle abduction palsy in one eye and limited adduction in the other eye. When you report your findings to the examiner, explain the movement's deficit rather than the cranial nerve. The terms hypertropia (pointing up), hypotropia (pointing down), esotropia (pointing inward) and exotropia (pointing outward) are useful. For example, a patient with an eye displaying esotropia or absence of abduction is called abduction palsy. This could originate from a VI cranial nerve palsy or mechanical reason in the orbit. A complete IIIrd cranial nerve palsy will result in a characteristic 'down and out' position in the affected eye. In IVth nerve palsy, patients report difficulty looking down when coming down a staircase.

INO, or the 'one and a half syndrome', which is more common in patients with multiple sclerosis, is a disorder of conjugate lateral gaze in which the affected eye shows impaired adduction. When an attempt is made to gaze contralaterally (relative to the affected eye), the affected eye adducts minimally, if at all. The contralateral eye abducts with nystagmus. Additionally, the divergence of the eyes leads to horizontal diplopia. Convergence is generally preserved. Be prepared to explain the anatomy of the medial longitudinal fasciculus.

Once you have detected a defect, perform further cranial nerve examinations. If you confirm an ophthalmoplegia, then examine the trigeminal nerve to exclude a possible cavernous sinus lesion.

If upward gaze is limited, examine for Parinaud's syndrome (dorsal midbrain syndrome). There will be abnormalities of eye movement and pupil function. The syndrome is characterized by a supranuclear vertical gaze paresis (upward more than downward), pseudo-Argyll Robertson pupils (accommodative paresis ensues, and the pupils become mid-dilated and show light-near dissociation), convergence-retraction nystagmus (nystagmus rectactorius), eyelid retraction (Collier's sign) and a conjugate downgaze in the neutral position ('setting-sun' sign).

If the examiner instructs you to examine the lower cranial nerves, decide whether you are just going to look at cranial nerves IX–XII or whether you also want to look at V–VIII depending on the clinical scenario.

Examination of the face

Examination of **cranial nerve V** is straightforward. The time taken for this examination is variable. The most sensitive test for cranial nerve V dysfunction is the loss of corneal reflex. (This is usually the only deficit even with a large trigeminal schwannoma.) In cases where you do not detect a blink reflex, ask the patient whether they can feel the stimulus. If the patient wears contact lenses, the blink reflex can be reduced. When testing the sensory branches of the cranial nerve V, it is important to apply the stimulus to each division (ophthalmic, maxillary and mandibular branches). For testing sensation in the maxillary division, apply the stimulus near the nasolabial fold or on the midline of the cheek. For testing sensation over the mandibular division, apply the stimulus on the anterior chin nearest to the midline. Avoid the skin over the angle of the mandible because this can also be supplied by the upper cervical cutaneous nerves. Examination of the motor component of cranial nerve V should be quick. Palpate for the contraction of the masseter and temporalis while the patient clenches the teeth, then assess lateral lower jaw movements against resistance (pterygoids). One can test the jaw jerk. Bear in mind the long length of the brainstem that contains the nuclei of the trigeminal nerve. It is also somatotopically arranged such that the most rostral parts supply the area around the nose and mouth and the more lateral areas are supplied by more caudal parts (e.g. like an onion skin).

Examination of **cranial nerve VII**: Initially, at rest, assess for any asymmetry, then ask the patient to perform the following manoeuvres: raise the eyebrows (frontalis muscle supplied by a temporal branch of the facial nerve), frown, close the eyes (orbicularis oculi) and blow out the cheeks and show the teeth (orbicularis oris). If a weakness is detected, be prepared to talk about the House–Brackmann grade and remember to inspect for a retrosigmoid scar. If the eye closure is incomplete, examine the corneal reflex (cranial nerve V). If both cranial V and VII are absent, one worries about corneal ulceration and a partial tarsorraphy ought to be considered. It is unlikely that you will be asked to formally assess taste but remember to at least ask about it.

Examination of **cranial nerve VIII** includes an assessment of hearing and balance. Begin by asking the patient if they have diminished hearing in one ear. Without this information, the interpretation of tuning fork tests will be complex. Inspect the ear canal and tympanic membrane to ensure that there is no obstruction or perforation. Use the appropriate tuning fork frequency (512/256 Hz) for the hearing tests. The tuning fork for vibration is 128 Hz.

Examination of **cranial nerves IX and X** is important. Glossopharyngeal nerve lesions can produce the following: difficulty swallowing; impairment of taste over the posterior one-third of the tongue and palate; impaired sensation over the posterior one-third of the tongue, palate and pharynx; an absent gag reflex and dysfunction of the parotid gland. Vagus nerve lesions produce palatal and pharyngeal paralysis;

laryngeal paralysis; abnormalities of oesophageal motility, gastric acid secretion, gallbladder emptying and heart rate; and other autonomic dysfunction. Begin by testing the patient's gag reflex. Remember this is an unpleasant test and the examiner may ask you to omit this. An absent gag reflex and/or deviation of the uvula (away from the side of the lesion) while asking the patient to say 'ah' indicate dysfunction of the IX–X cranial nerves. If the gag reflex is absent, assess if the patient has preserved sensation on both sides of the oropharynx. Occasionally, patients who have worn dentures for a long time may lose the gag reflex, although the pharyngeal sensation remains intact. Ask the patient to cough and note if a hoarse voice is present. If the latter sign is present, consider a further assessment by formal laryngoscopy.

Examination of **cranial nerve XI** assesses the actions of trapezius and sternocleido-mastoid muscles. Observe the volume and contour of the sternocleidomastoid muscles as the patient looks straight ahead. Test the right sternocleidomastoid muscle by facing the patient and placing your right palm laterally on the patient's left cheek. Ask the patient to turn the head to the left, resisting the pressure you are exerting in the opposite direction. At the same time, observe and palpate the right sternoclei-domastoid with your left hand. Then reverse the procedure to test the left sternoclei-domastoid. Now test the trapezius muscle. Ask the patient to face away from you. Observe the shoulder contour for hollowing, displacement or winging of the scapula and drooping of the shoulder. Place your hands on the patient's shoulders and press down as the patient shrugs the shoulders and then retracts.

The examination of **cranial nerve XII** starts by inspecting the tongue with the opened mouth while the tongue remains within the oral cavity. Fasciculations are reliably detected before tongue protrusion. If there is cranial nerve palsy on protruding the tongue, it becomes deviated toward the side of a lesion as a result of the weakness of the action of the genioglossus muscle. Movements from side to side against the resis-tance of the cheeks would detect more subtle weakness. If there is a significant weak-ness, assess for hemiatrophy, which reflects the longstanding nature of this deficit.

Summary of cranial nerve (I–XII) examination

I Olfactory

Assess the patient's sense of smell by testing each nostril in turn. Use essence bottles of coffee, vanilla and peppermint.

II Optic

General: Observe for pupil asymmetry, ptosis and swelling.

Visual acuity: If the patient wears glasses, keep them on. Test each eye separately using a Snellen chart.

Visual fields: Stand 2 feet in front of the patient and ensure that you are at eye level. Move your hands to the side halfway between yourself and the patient, wiggle fingers and ask the patient when they see movement. Assess nasal and temporal fields.

Fundoscopy: Assess the fundus, macula and optic disc.

III, IV and VI Oculomotor, Trochlear and Abducens

Inspect the pupils and look for ptosis: Shape and presence of ptosis.

Pupil reaction: To light (direct, consensual and swinging light test) and accommodation.

Extra-ocular eye movements:
Assess saccadic and pursuit eye movements.

V Trigeminal

Facial sensation: Forehead, cheek and jaw.

Motor: Assess the following muscles: Temporalis, masseter, pterygoids.

Ask the patient to open their mouth and clench their teeth.

Assess bite strength.

Assess corneal reflex.

Assess jaw jerk.

VII Facial

Inspect for facial droop or asymmetry.

Facial expression: Ask the patient to look up and wrinkle their forehead. Inspect for wrinkle loss. Ask the patient to shut their eyes tightly. Ask the patient to smile and look for asymmetry in the patient's nasolabial folds. In addition, ask the patient to frown, show their teeth and puff out their cheeks. Assess for taste.

VIII Vestibulocochlear

Auditory acuity of each ear: Place your hands by each of the patient's ears. Rub your fingers to create noise on one side and keep the other hand still. Then switch hands. Ask the patient from which ear the noise is heard. If hearing loss is identified, inspect the external auditory canals and the tympanic membranes.

Rinne's test (air vs. bone conduction).

Apply the tuning fork (512/256 Hz) to the mastoid behind the ear. Ask the patient when they can no longer hear the sound. Then move the tuning fork next to the patient's ear canal so they can hear the sound. A normal response is that air conduction (ear) is better heard than bone conduction (mastoid).

Weber's test (lateralization).

Apply a tuning fork to the top of patient's head on the middle of the forehead. Ask the patient 'where do you hear the sound coming from?' A normal response is in the midline.

Test oculocephalic reflex (doll's eye manoeuvre).

Test oculovestibular reflex (ear canal caloric stimulation) - only in brainstem death testing.

IX and X Glossopharygeal, Vagus

Assess the patient's voice for hoarseness.

Ask the patient to swallow and cough.

Examine the palate for uvular displacement.

Assess the soft palate movement by asking the patient to say 'ah'.

Perform the gag reflex.

XI Accessory

Examine for atrophy and asymmetry of the trapezius and sternocleidomastoid muscle.

Ask the patient to shrug their shoulders.

Turn the patient's head against resistance, inspect and palpate the sternocleidomastoid muscle.

XII Hypoglossal

Listen to articulation.

Inspect the patient's tongue for wasting or fasciculations.

Ask the patient to protrude the tongue: The tongue will deviate to the affected side.

The timing and speed of your cranial nerve examination is key. A slow examination results in a missed opportunity to examine other clinical cases and gives the impression that you are inexperienced and lack confidence. A hasty examination may result in the omission of key important signs.

7 Cerebellar evaluation

The cerebellum coordinates the unconscious regulation of balance, muscle tone and coordination of voluntary movement.

Cerebellar dysfunction is assessed by using the mnemonic DANISH

- **D**ysdiadochokinesia. Ask the patient to rapidly pronate and supinate their hand on the opposite side. Repeat with the other hand. The patient will have an inability to perform rapid alternating movements.
- **A**taxia. Assess for a broad-based unsteady gait with lumbering movements. The patient may demonstrate the variable distance between steps and difficulty with turning.
- **N**ystagmus. Assess for oscillating eye movements.
- **I**ntention tremor. Ask the patient to point from their nose to your finger. Ensure that your finger is at arm's length and then move your finger to different places. As the patient's finger approaches your finger, a tremor may be noticed or there may be evidence of past pointing.
- **S**taccato speech. Ask the patient to repeat 'British constitution' or 'pink hippopotamus'.
- **H**ypotonia. Assess for reduced tone in the patient's upper and lower limbs.

Remember that cerebellar dysfunction may coexist with lower cranial nerve dysfunction. If there is time, one should go through at least CN IX–XII if not V–XII. The location of posterior fossa scars can be particularly helpful.

8 Gait evaluation

- **Walking**: Initiation, gait symmetry, size of paces, posture, arms swing, turning, speed, fluency of stepping, stride length and distance between feet (base). Also, inspect the patient's knees, pelvis and shoulders.
- **Inspect the patient's shoes**.
- **Ask the patient to heel-to-toe walk (as if on a tightrope), walk on their toes and heels**.
- **Romberg test** (to assess the dorsal columns of the spinal cord): Ask the patient to stand with the feet together and close their eyes.

9 Peripheral nervous system evaluation (upper and lower limbs)

It may seem an obvious thing to say, but one must decide on what the focus of the examination is – brain, cord, nerve root or peripheral nerve. An arm weakness following resection of GBM will need a different examination from a patient with radial nerve palsy following fracture of the humerus. A brain lesion will generally result in hemibody dysfunction coexisting with upper motor neurone signs – pronator drift is useful. A cord dysfunction will result in a motor and sensory level with long tract signs (again UMN). A root problem will affect a dermatome and a myotome. For peripheral nerve dysfunction, one will need to know the specific muscles supplied and the area of sensation. For cord and root problems, we would recommend going through the examination as detailed in the American Spinal Injuries Association (ASIA) chart. This provides a very reproducible and systematic way of examining sensation and power in upper and lower limbs. When there is no clue as to the anatomical origin, again, the ASIA chart approach tends to be safe (Figure 2.3).

Upper limb examination

- Introduce and ask permission to examine the patient.
- Expose the upper limbs.
- Comment on the patient's surroundings (hand splints, medication).
- Detailed inspection.
  - Inspect the patient as a whole (posture/cachectic/pain-free/in pain).
  - Inspect for the following: Asymmetry, deformities, scars, tremor, muscle wasting, fasciculations, involuntary movements, peripheral stigmata of underlying neurological disease and supraclavicular fullness. Remember scars may well be in the neck (anterior or posterior).
- Muscle tone.
  - Ask the patient whether there is any pain.
  - Take the patient by the hand in a 'hand shake' and support the elbow with your other hand. In turn test each joint, in particular supination/pronation and wrist movement.
  - Remember the differences between rigidity and spasticity.

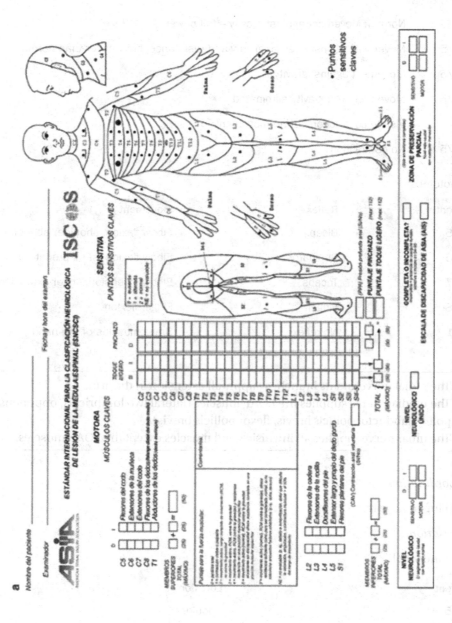

Figure 2.3 American Spinal Cord Injury Association (ASIA) Impairemnet Scale

Table of spasticity and rigidity

Power

- Ask the patient to raise the arms. Comment on evidence of a pronator drift or limb weakness

MRC Grade

5/5	Normal: Movement against gravity – full power
4/5	Movement against specific gravity and resistance, but weaker than normal
3/5	Movement against gravity
2/5	Movement with gravity eliminated
1/5	Visible contraction but no movement
0/5	No contraction

Myotomes

Root	Reflex	Movement
C5	Biceps	Elbow flexion, shoulder abduction
C6	Supinator	Elbow flexion (semi pronated)
C7	Triceps	Elbow extension, finger extension
C8	Finger	Finger flexion
T1	No reflex	Small muscles of the hand

- The radial nerve and its branches supply all extension in the arm.
- The median nerve supplies the LOAF muscles (lateral two lumbricals, opponens pollics, abductor pollicis brevis, flexor pollicis brevis).
- The ulnar nerve supplies all intrinsic hand muscles except the LOAF muscles.

Coordination

- Finger–nose test.

Sensation

- Fine touch.

Root	Location
C5	Shoulder
C6	Lateral arm/thumb
C7	Back of hand
C8	Medial hand
T1	Medial arm

- Pinprick.
- Temperature.
- Two-point discrimination.
- Joint position sense (shoulder, elbow, finger).
- Vibration sense (sternum, wrist, elbow, shoulder) - use 128Hz tuning fork.

Reflexes

- Biceps (C5, C6).
- Supinator (C5, C6).
- Triceps (C6, C7).
- Finger flexors – Hoffmann's sign.
- Pectoral reflex.
- Deltoid reflex.

Reflexes are graded using a 0 to 4+ scale.

Grade	Description
0	Absent
+	Hypoactive
++	Normal
+++	Hyperactive without clonus
++++	Hyperactive with clonus

Complete the upper limb examination

- Examine the patient's spine.
- Examine the cranial nerves and neurology of the lower limbs.

Arrange for appropriate investigations

- Bedside tests (e.g. observation charts, dipstick urine, ECG).
- Bloods (e.g. group and save, FBC, U&E, CRP).
- Radiological imaging (e.g. radiographs, CT scan and MRI scan).
- Special tests (e.g. EEG, nerve conduction studies, PET scan).

Treatment options

- Conservative.
- Medical.
- Radiological.
- Surgical.

Lower limb examination

- Introduce yourself and ask permission to examine patient.
- Ask if the patient would mind exposing their lower limbs.
- Comment on the patient's surroundings (leg splints, medication).
- Detailed inspection.

- Inspect the patient as a whole (e.g. well/unwell/cachectic/pain-free/in pain).
- Inspect for the following:
  - Asymmetry, deformities, scars, tremor, muscle wasting, fasciculations and involuntary movements, peripheral stigmata of underlying neurological disease.
  - Assess the back for deformity or scars.
- Gait.
  - Perform Romberg's test. Ask the patient to walk to a fixed point, walk heel – toe and walk on heels and toes.
  - Inspect patient's shoes.
  - Comment on the patient's posture.
- Muscle tone.
  - Ask the patient whether there is any pain.
  - Roll the legs, lift and release the knees. Assess for rigidity.
  - Test for clonus.
  - Test plantars.
- Power.
  - Ask the patient to lift the legs. Comment on the evidence of limb weakness.

MRC Grade

5/5	Normal: movement against gravity – full power
4/5	Movement against specific gravity and resistance but weaker than normal
3/5	Movement against gravity
2/5	Movement with gravity eliminated
1/5	Visible contraction but no movement
0/5	No contraction

Myotomes

Root	Reflex	Movement
L1,L2	No reflex	Hip flexion
L3,L4	Knee reflex	Knee extension
L5	No reflex	Dorsiflexion of foot, inversion and eversion of ankle, extension of great toe
S1	Ankle reflex	Hip extension, knee extension, plantarflexion

Coordination

- Heel-shin test.

Sensation

- Fine touch.

Root	Location
L1	Inguinal area
L2,3	Anterior thigh
L4	Medial malleolus
L5	Dorsum of foot
S1	Lateral foot and sole

- Pinprick.
- Temperature.
- Two-point discrimination.
- Joint position sense (hip, knee, toes).
- Vibration sense (ankle, tibial tuberosity, iliac crest).

Reflexes

- Knee (L3, L4).
- Ankle (L5, S1).
- Plantar reflex: Babinski (extensor).

Reflexes are graded using a 0 to 4+ scale.

Grade	Description
0	Absent
+	Hypoactive
++	Normal
+++	Hyperactive without clonus
++++	Hyperactive with clonus

Complete the lower limb examination.

- Examine the patient's spine. Look for scars!
- Examine the cranial nerves and neurology of the upper limbs.

Arrange for appropriate investigations.

- Bedside tests (e.g. observation charts, dipstick urine, ECG).
- Bloods (e.g. Group and Save, FBC, U&E, CRP).
- Radiological imaging (e.g. Radiographs, CT scan and MRI scan).
- Special tests (e.g. EEG, nerve conduction studies, PET scan).

Treatment options.

- Conservative.
- Medical.
- Radiological.
- Surgical.

10 Paediatric history and examination evaluation

There are fundamental differences between infants or young children and adolescents or adults as far as neurological examination is concerned.

History: Obtaining a good history is crucial and it requires good rapport between the physician, the child and the family. The child should be encouraged to express and describe symptoms with its own words. History should include the following:

1. **History of presenting complaint**
   a. Onset, duration, pattern, modifying factors, associated symptoms and localization of the symptoms.
   b. Establish prior baseline function.
   c. Is there underlying inherited disease?
   d. Is there underlying metabolic disorder?
2. **Birth history**
   a. **Antenatal course**: Determine if there was a natural conception or achieved through assisted reproductive technology. Maternal factors should also be determined such as age, past medical history (e.g. diabetes), history of infections (TORCHS, LCMV, HPV, HIV) and history of drugs or toxins exposure.
   b. **Labour and delivery**: Mode of delivery and use of aids in case of vaginal delivery should be known, gestational age (extremely preterm <28 weeks, preterm 28–34 weeks, late preterm 34–36 weeks, term 37–42 weeks), APGAR score and birth weight as well as growth chart should be checked.
   c. **Postnatal course**: Postnatal complication should be considered. For example mechanical ventilation, sepsis, hypoglycaemia and history of neonatal seizures should be documented. History of neonatal seizures, especially the first 12–24 hours may be indicative of hypoxic-ischaemic encephalopathy.
3. **Developmental history**
   a. Abnormal patterns provide information regarding the child's underlying neurological disorder.
   b. Developmental milestones may be separated into four functional areas:
      i. Gross motor.
      ii. Vision and fine motor.
      iii. Hearing, speech and language.
      iv. Social, emotional and behavioural.
   c. A delay should be classified as mild, moderate or severe according to the deviation from normal.
   d. Of note, the developmental milestones should be corrected with regards to the gestational age and prematurity.
   e. Regression of the skills may also occur and may underline neurodegenerative disease.
4. **Past medical and surgical history**
5. **Family and social history**
   a. Autosomal, X-linked and mitochondrial inheritance patterns should be considered.
   b. Social and environmental factors may also contribute to significant neurological manifestation.

Examination

1. Dysmorphology.
   a. Genetic syndromes have specific patterns expressed.
2. Neurocutaneous stigmata.
   a. There is known association between neurocutaneous lesion and central nervous system (CNS) abnormalities.
   b. Check for skin colour pigmentation or discolouration.
   c. Neuro-axis should also be checked for dimples or tuft of hair. These finding are indicative of spina bifida.
3. Head size and shape.
   a. Measuring and plotting the occipital frontal circumference (OFC) is essential essence. The OFC is measured over the most prominent part of the back of the head (occiput) and just above the eyebrow (supraorbital ridges). Microcephaly and macrocephaly may be indicative of underlying structural abnormalities. Of note, parents' head size and shape should be considered.
   b. Abnormalities of skull shapes should be documented and craniosynostosis should be ruled out.
   c. Anterior fontanelle typically closes between 12th and 18th week. Premature fusion of the anterior fontanelle should raise suspicion of microcephaly or craniosynostosis. On the other hand, persistence of the anterior fontanelle beyond the 18th week may indicate raised ICP or hypothyroidism.
4. Paediatric Glasgow Coma Score.
   - Eyes
     - E4 Spontaneous
     - E3 To voice
     - E2 To pain
     - E1 None
     - C Eyes closed (e.g. bandage, swelling)
   - Verbal
     - V5 Alert, babbles, coos, words or sentences to usual ability (normal) orientated
     - V4 Cries, irritable but consolable confused
     - V3 Cries to pain, occasionally consolable inappropriate words
     - V2 Moans to pain, inconsolable, agitated incomprehensible sounds
     - V1 None
     - T Intubated
   - Motor
     - M6 Normal spontaneous movements obeys commands
     - M5 Localizes to pain
     - M4 Flexion – withdrawal
     - M3 Flexion – abnormal (decorticate rigidity)
     - M2 Extension (decerebrate rigidity)
     - M1 No response
5. Primitive reflexes: Of note, most of the primitive reflexes are present in utero and regress within the first 6–12 months of age. Retention of the reflexes may underline neurological disorder and can be related to future developmental delays.
   Primitive reflex appearance of the reflex disappearance of the reflex

- Moro   birth 4–6 months
- Tonic labyrinthine   birth 3–3.5 years
- Asymmetrical tonic neck reflex   birth 3 months
- Symmetrical tonic neck reflex   3 months 10–12 months
- Palmar/Plantar grasp   birth 3–6 months/6–8 months
- Rooting   birth 3–4 months
- Spinal gallant   birth 2 months
- Suck/swallow   birth 18 months/persists voluntarily
- Babinski   birth 2 years
- Stepping and placing   birth persists voluntarily
- Parachute   birth 8 months
- Landau   2–3 months 6 months
- Babkin   birth 4 months

6. Cranial nerves.
   a. CN I (Olfactory): Rarely tested in children except when anosmia is an important consideration.
   b. CN II (Optic): Visual acuity, visual fields, pupillary light reflex and fundoscopic examination. Confrontational visual field examination in a young child is challenging if not impossible. However, a blink response to a threat provides a gross assessment of visual field integrity.
   c. CN III, IV and VI (Oculomotor, Trochlear, Abducens): The use of bright, colourful objects in an infant or young child is essential in order to gain attention.
   d. CN V (Trigeminal): The rooting reflex in the neonate can provide a crude assessment of nerve function.
   e. CN VII (Facial): The facial nerve can be tested in babies by direct observation when feeding or crying. In older children, the nerve is tested by asking them to make 'funny faces'.
   f. CN VIII (Vestibulocochlear): A neonate will alert and quieten to a bell presented at their ear. By the age of 6 months, the baby will turn and localize the sound if hearing is intact.
   g. CV IX and X (Glossopharyngeal and Vagus): Eliciting gag response, especially in babies, is often necessary to assess palatal function.
   h. CN XI (Accessory). Look for shoulder movements.
   i. CN XII (Hypoglossal): In neonate, hypoglossal nerve can be tested by placing a finger in the mouth and appreciating the movements of the tongue.
7. Motor examination
   a. Pyramidal, extrapyramidal and cerebellar systems should be tested.
   b. Muscle bulk, tone and power are required to be documented.
      i. Check for muscle atrophy, asymmetry or hypertrophy.
      ii. Check for fasciculations.
      iii. Check for muscle tenderness.
      iv. Muscle tone should be differentiated between spasticity and rigidity.
      v. Of note, spasticity typically develops the first year of life as the nerve system matures.
      vi. Check for hand preference in early life. This may indicate weakness given that hand preference before the age of 12–18 months old is considered abnormal.

      vii. Cerebellar function is challenging to test in babies and young children; however, through games it can be effectively checked. Test for truncal ataxia and gait via observation whilst the patient is playing.

  c. Involuntary movements

      i. Look for hyperkinetic movements such as chorea, athetosis, tremors, ballismus, dystonia, tics and myclonus.

      ii. Hypokinetic movements include bradykinesia, akinesia or rigidity.

8. Sensory examination.

  a. It is the most challenging part of neurologically examination. Though complete sensory examination is required, including light touch, pain and temperature, proprioception and vibration, as well as graphesthesia, two-point discrimination and stereognosis.

  b. Babies can be tested for light touch and pain by watching their facial response and grimacing.

  c. In older children, sensory examination findings can be inconsistent and thus repetition may be needed.

11 Parkinson's disease patient evaluation

It is not necessarily a routine examination for most trainees but can come up in a clinical on deep brain stimulation. As examiners may ask about functional neurosurgery, a hot topic is deep brain stimulation.

- *Inspection*: Lack of facial expression, reduced spontaneous movements, reduced blinking, tremor at rest – pill rolling (4–6 Hz), stooped posture.
- *Speech*: Hypophonia.
- *Bradykinesia*: Rapid alternating movements – tapping thumb and index finger, fist open/close, pronation/supination of hand, toe tapping and heel tapping.
- *Rigidity*: Assess with the circling movement of wrist and elbow. Distracting manoeuvres such as asking the patient to tap their other knee can bring out subtle rigidity.
- *Tremor*: Resting, postural (put hands outstretched) and action tremor (finger nose test).
- *Gait and balance*: The ability to stand from seated without using arms, observation of gait (shuffling, heel strike, arm swing). Pull test.
- *Special tests*: Assessment of writing and glabellar tap (not approved by some neurologists).

12 Neurocutaneous syndrome evaluation

These syndromes are a favourite for professional examinations. The diagnosis is made on clinical history and examination and confirmed by diagnostic testing. The most common types of neurocutaneous syndromes are the following:

1. Tuberous sclerosis
2. Neurofibromatosis (1 and 2)
3. Von Hippel-Lindau disease
4. Struge-Weber syndrome
5. Osler-Weber-Rendu syndrome

1 Tuberous sclerosis: Clinical presentation

A 23-year-old man presents with a 3-year history of headaches, which have progressed over the past 1–2 months. In addition, he presents with symptoms of nausea and vomiting. His past medical history includes seizures, which resolved when he was 10 years of age.

Tuberous sclerosis is a rare multisystem genetic disease (autosomal dominant) characterized by hamartomas of many organs including skin, brain, eyes, kidneys, heart and lungs. The combination of symptoms includes seizures, intellectual disability, developmental delay, behavioural problems, skin abnormalities and diseases of the lung and kidney. It is caused by mutation of either of two genes, *TSC1* (chromosome 9) and *TSC2* (chromosome 16), which code for the proteins hamartin and tuberin, respectively. These proteins act as tumour growth suppressors.

The classic clinical triad consists of seizures, mental retardation and sebaceous adenomas.

Patients present with the following:

- Facial angiofibromas.
- Periungual and subungal fibromas.
- Fibrous plaques of the forehead and scalp.

Associated conditions:

- Tubers.
- Subependymal giant cell astrocytoma (SEGA).
- Multiple calcified subependymal nodules.
- Multiple retinal astrocytomas.
- Retinal hamartomas or achromic patch.
- Shagreen patch.
- Pulmonary lymphangiomyomatosis.
- Renal angiomyolipoma.
- Renal cysts.
- Cardiac rhabdomyomas.

2 Neurofibromatosis (1 and 2): Clinical presentation

A 29-year-old left-handed woman presents with unilateral hearing loss and tinnitus. Moreover, she presents with reduced visual acuity and diplopia.

Neurofibromatosis (NF) refers to a number of inherited conditions that are clinically and genetically distinct and carry a high risk of tumour formation, particularly in the brain. Neurofibromatosis is an autosomal dominant condition. The severity in affected individuals can vary; this may be due to variable expression. Approximately half of the cases are due to *de novo* mutations and no other affected family members are seen.

Neurofibromatosis 1 (>90% of cases of neurofibromatosis), chromosome 17q11.2, which codes for neurofibromin.

1. Six or more café-au-lait spots (≥ 0.5 cm in prepubertal subjects or ≥ 1.5 cm in postpuberta subjects).
2. ≥ 2 neurofibromas or one plexiform neurofibroma.
3. Freckling in the axilla or groin.
4. Optic glioma.
5. Two or more Lisch nodules.
6. A distinctive bony lesion (dysplasia of the sphenoid bone or dysplasia or thinning of long bone cortex).
7. A first-degree relative with NF-1.

Associated conditions

- Schwann cell tumours on any nerve.
- Spinal +/− peripheral nerve neurofibromas.
- Multiple skin neurofibromas.
- Aqueductal stenosis.
- Macrocephaly.
- Intracranial tumours: astroctyomas and mengingiomas.
- Optic glioma.
- Kyphoscoliosis.
- Syringomyelia.
- Malignant tumours: neuroblastoma, ganglioma, sarcoma, leukaemia and Wilm's tumour.
- Phaechromocytoma.
- Mental retardation.
- Learning difficulties.

Neurofibromatosis 2, chromosome 22q12.2, which results in the inactivation of schwannomin.

1. Bilateral vestibular schwannomas.
2. OR first-degree relative with NF-2 and either:
   A. Unilateral eight nerve mass.
   B. OR two of the following:
      1. Neurofibroma.
      2. Meningioma.
      3. Glioma: Includes astrocytoma, ependymoma.
      4. Schwannomas: Including spinal root schwannoma.
      5. Juvenile posterior subcapsular lenticular opacities or cataract.

Associated conditions include the following:

- Seizures.
- Skin nodules, dermal neurofibromas, café au lait spots (less common than NF-1).
- Multiple intradural spinal tumours (less common in NF-1) including intramedullary (ependymomas) and extramedullary (schwannomas, meningioma) tumours.
- Antigenic nerve growth factor is increased.

3 Von Hippel–Lindau disease: Clinical presentation

A 36-year-old man presents with nausea, vomiting and headaches for 1 week. His MRI scan demonstrates a dilated fourth ventricle with a cystic lesion in the left cerebellar hemisphere.

VHL disease is a rare autosomal dominant genetic condition that predisposes individuals to benign and malignant tumours. VHL results from a mutation in the VHL tumour suppressor gene on chromosome 3p25.3.

1. One or more haemangioblastomas (HGBs) within the CNS (typically a cerebellar HGB and a retinal HGB and angioma).
2. Inconstant presence of visceral lesions (usually renal +/– pancreatic tumours or cysts).
3. Frequent familial incidence.

Associated conditions

- HGBs of the cerebellum and spinal cord.
- Retinal angiomas.
- Retinal HGBs.
- Renal cell carcinomas.
- Pheochromocytomas.
- Polycythemia.
- Cysts (hepatic, renal, pancreas and epididymal).
- Endolymphatic sac tumour.
- Epididymal papillary cystadenomas.

4 Sturge–Weber syndrome: Clinical presentation

A 34-year-old man presents with a grand mal seizure while at work. He suffers from long-standing epilepsy and headaches.

Sturge–Weber syndrome is a rare congenital neurological and skin disorder. It is often associated with port-wine stains of the face, glaucoma, seizures, mental retardation and ipsilateral leptomeningeal angioma. It is characterized by abnormal blood vessels on the brain surface. Normally, only one side of the brain is affected. Sturge–Weber is an embryonal developmental anomaly resulting from errors in mesodermal and ectodermal development. Most cases are sporadic. It is caused by a somatic activating mutation occurring in the GNAQ gene.

A. Localized cerebral cortical atrophy and calcifications (especially layers 2 and 3, with a predilection for the occipital lobes):
    1. Calcifications appear as curvilinear double parallel lines ('tram tracking') on plain X-rays.
    2. Cortical atrophy usually causes contralateral haemiparesis, haemiatrophy and homonymous haemianopia (with occipital lobe involvement).
B. Ipsilateral port-wine facial nevus (nevus fammeus) usually in the distribution of the ophthalmic division of trigeminal nerve).

Associated conditions

- Ipsilateral exophthalmos +/− glaucoma, coloboma of the iris.
- Oculomeningeal capillary haemangioma.
- Convulsive seizures (contralateral to the facial nevus and cortical atrophy).
- Retinal angioma.
- Haemiparesis.
- Mental retardation.
- Learning disability.
- Developmental delay.
- Haemianopsia.
- Vascular headaches.
- Moyamoya disease.
- AVMs of the lung and liver.

5 Osler–Weber–Rendu syndrome: Clinical presentation

A 53-year-old woman presents with recurrent epistaxis, which requires repeated hospital admissions.

Osler–Weber–Rendu syndrome (hereditary haemorrhagic telangiectasia [HHT]) is a rare autosomal dominant genetic disorder that is linked to tumour growth factor B (TGF-B), HHTL (endoglin, chromosome 9) and HHT2 (ALK1, chromosome 12). Haploinsufficiency leads to a deficiency in angiogenesis. This leads to abnormal blood vessel formation in the skin, in the mucous membranes and often in organs such as the lungs, liver and brain.

Associated conditions

- Recurrent epistaxis.
- Cerebrovascular malformations including telangiectasia, AVMs, venous angiomas and aneurysms.
- Pulmonary arteriovenous fistulas with risk of paradoxical cerebral embolism, which predisposes to embolic stroke and cerebral abscess.

Summary and Advise

- Be aware of the total duration allotted for this section and the minimal time required for an individual case as this may vary slightly from one case to another. For example, a spot case of an acromegaly may take 1–2 minutes only for discussion as compared to taking a focused history of someone with a seizure.
- Relax, stand back and listen to the instructions given by the examiners carefully. Listen to the clues given.
- Do not hurry to get close or touch the patient. Take a step back and inspect the patient from afar as this manoeuvre may give you a clue to the type of case you are dealing with. Remember 'He who is in a hurry arrives late'.
- Use medical terminology during your discussion of the case with your examiners. Precise usage of terminology will reduce ambiguity and will reflect well on you as a 'Day One Consultant'.

- **Examiners are there to help you. Therefore, help them by not antagonizing them.**
- **Once you have finished with one station, and before moving on to the next, it is important to remain calm and collected. Try to 'block off' any bad memories from the preceding station. Treat each station as an individual examination.**

3 The Viva: Operative Surgery and Surgical Anatomy

We intend to guide you through the examination questions that are considered 'favourites'. It is important to couple this revision guide with neurosurgical operative textbooks. In this section of the examination, the examiner assesses your surgical anatomy, knowledge and how you avoid potential surgical complications. Therefore, it must be stressed that the main emphasis is on the surgical anatomy of the approach and complication avoidance. During the operative surgery and surgical anatomy Viva, we recommend that you convey your personal experience rather than reciting a surgical textbook. Throughout this chapter, short tables are added to identify important key points and potential challenging areas of discussion. The selected procedures are not an exhaustive list, but rather demonstrate common principles that can be applied in presenting a variety of operations in the examination setting. For some important procedures, the emphasis is on the surgical principles and specific points that are likely to be asked. This is to remind the reader that it is important to understand the basic principles of surgical adjuncts (e.g. technical equipment and instruments, intraoperative dyes, neurophysiological intraoperative monitoring, angiographic planning in vascular cases, special anaesthetic techniques) because they are likely to be assessed. For specialized or uncommon operations, examiners tend to focus on specific essential points. The candidate must remain calm (and not panic) when asked about these rare operations because it is not the technical details that the examiners want to hear, but rather they would like to assess the candidate's understanding of the basic principles.

Standard operations

If you are asked about a standard operation, then it is best to provide a clear answer emphasizing three key points in the allocated time. For these types of questions, it is important to communicate the operative steps. The discussion begins in the preoperative period by confirming the diagnosis, obtaining informed consent and marking the patient. Safety and the avoidance of complications are key. When possible, describe the operation in terms of relevant anatomy. Avoid prolonged narratives of minor steps. The operative steps should be described in a way indicating your personal surgical experience and not from an operative textbook. For example, if you are asked to perform anterior cervical decompression and fusion (ACDF), then it is expected that you will describe the whole procedure from start to finish in the allocated time. No prompting should be required. Please ensure that you localize the

DOI: 10.1201/9781003254379-3

correct level and avoid injury to the surrounding structures (e.g. pharynx, oesophagus, trachea, recurrent laryngeal nerve injury and spinal cord).

Complex operations

If you are asked about a complex operation, then it is best to start the discussion with the required pre-operative investigations, alternative treatments, surgical indications and informed consent (with the benefits and potential risks of surgery). It is important to discuss the key salient features and that you would involve the multidisciplinary team (MDT), when appropriate. The reason for these questions is to test your neuroanatomy knowledge and to see if you are aware of potential complications leading to post-operative morbidity and mortality.

For example, if you are asked to debulk a pineal tumour, it is important to confirm the diagnosis with the appropriate radiological imaging and evaluate serum and cerebrospinal fluid (CSF) tumour markers. Include the management of hydrocephalus if present. Treatment includes close observation while awaiting surgery, external ventricular drainage (EVD), endoscopic third ventriculostomy (ETV) ± biopsy or insertion of a ventricular peritoneal (VP) shunt. When asked to describe the operative steps, mention anatomical landmarks and key safety points. Mention the common approaches (e.g. infratentorial supracerebellar, occipital transtentorial and transcallosal interhemispheric), preservation of the deep venous system (internal cerebral veins, vein of Galen and basal vein of Rosenthal) and avoidance of a complete tumour resection if the midbrain tectum is grossly infiltrated.

Moreover, it is important to familiarize yourself with the 'tools' used during neurosurgical operations. Key topics include CUSA (cavitron ultrasonic surgical aspirator), microscopic-integrated ICG (IndoCyanine Green), high-speed drills, neuronavigation and 5-ALA (5-aminolevulinic acid) fluorescence-guided surgery.

Anatomical landmarks

With an emphasis on neuroanatomy, cranio-cerebral relationships are frequently asked. The following are key favourite anatomical landmarks.

Central sulcus

The central sulcus is an anatomical landmark along a straight line from a point midway between the lateral canthus and ear canal (or from a point about 5 cm straight up from the ear canal) to a point about 2 cm posterior to the mid-distance between the nasion and inion in the midline. This makes the motor cortex more or less in line with the ear canal near the midline or about 4–5 cm posterior to the coronal suture.

Calcarine fissure

The calcarine fissure is an anatomical landmark located at the caudal end of the medial surface of the brain. The calcarine sulcus begins near the occipital pole in two converging rami and runs forward to a point a little below the splenium of the corpus callosum, where it is joined at an acute angle by the medial part of the parieto-occipital sulcus. The anterior part of this fissure gives rise to the prominence of the calcar avis in the posterior cornu of the lateral ventricle.

Foramen of Monro

The foramen of Monro connects the paired lateral ventricles with the third ventricle at the midline of the brain. The trajectory to the foramen is in line with the coronal suture (as it meets the superior temporal line).

Lateral limb of the Sylvian fissure

The lateral limb of the Sylvian fissure lies along a line connecting the lateral canthus to three-quarters the distance between the nasion and inion in the midline.

Parieto-occipital sulcus

The lateral part of the sulcus is situated about 5 cm in front of the occipital pole. The medial part runs downward and forward as a deep cleft on the medial surface of the hemisphere and joins the calcarine fissure below and behind the posterior end of the corpus callosum. In most cases, it contains a submerged gyrus. It marks the boundary between the cuneus and precuneus and also between the parietal and occipital lobes. It is located approximately in line with the lambdoid suture.

Transverse sinus

The transverse sinuses are of large size and begin at the internal occipital protuberance; one, generally the right, being the direct continuation of the superior sagittal sinus (SSS), the other the continuation of the straight sinus. They drain from the confluence of sinuses to the sigmoid sinuses, which ultimately connect to the internal jugular vein. They can be marked on the skin along the line connecting the inion and root of zygoma. The important angle where transverse becomes sigmoid sinus lies where the vertical line from the digastric notch of the mastoid meets the inion-zygoma line. This should be in the region of the asterion, although this can be a variable guide.

Further examples of important intracranial landmarks

Anterior ethmoidal foramen

The anterior ethmoidal foramen is a small opening formed when the anterior ethmoidal notch on the superior margin of the ethmoid bone corresponds to a similar small notch in the frontal bone creating a small foramen in the sutural junction of the two bones. The foramen transmits the anterior ethmoidal nerve, a branch of the nasociliary nerve, into the anterior and middle ethmoidal sinuses and nasal cavity. It also indicates the anterior extent of the cribriform plate. Identification of the anterior ethmoidal artery is an important landmark in endonasal endoscopic surgery as it passes from the orbit to anterior cranial fossa.

Arcuate eminence

This is a distinct, rounded prominence on the superior surface of the petrous temporal bone. It sits about halfway between the petrosquamous suture and the apex of the bone. This rounded eminence marks the position of the anterior semicircular canal in the inner ear.

First denticulate ligament

The denticulate ligament is located in the pia mater of the spinal cord. It attaches the pia mater to the arachnoid and dura maters. The first ligament separates the spinal accessory nerve (which is the only motor root that is dorsal to the denticulate ligaments) from the vertebral artery.

Flocculus

The flocculus is the smallest lobe of the cerebellum. It is located at the anterior part of the hemisphere, between the biventral lobe and the middle peduncle of the cerebellum, in the line of the horizontal fissure. Boundaries: inferior to cranial nerves VII/VIII and superior to cranial nerves IX/X/XI.

Frontal horn of the lateral ventricle

The frontal horn is a portion of the lateral ventricle that passes forward and laterally, from the interventricular foramen to the frontal lobe, curving around the anterior end of the caudate nucleus. Its floor is formed by the upper surface of the reflected portion of the corpus callosum, the rostrum. It is bounded medially by the anterior portion of the septum pellucidum and laterally by the head of the caudate nucleus. Its apex reaches the posterior surface of the genu of the corpus callosum. It is located deep in the inferior frontal gyrus.

Temporal horn of the lateral ventricle

The temporal horn traverses the temporal lobe of the brain, forming in its course a curve around the posterior end of the thalamus. Its floor is composed of the hippocampus, the fimbria hippocampi, the collateral eminence, and the choroid plexus. Its roof is formed chiefly by the inferior surface of the tapetum of the corpus callosum, but the tail of the caudate nucleus and the stria terminalis also extend forward in the roof of the inferior cornu to its extremity; the tail of the caudate nucleus joins the putamen. It is located deep in the middle temporal gyrus.

The choroid fissure is C-shaped around the thalamus with the outside limit being the tail of hippocampus and fornix. The inferior choroidal point is in the temporal horn, and choroidal branches from the anterior choroidal and lateral posterior choroidal arteries supplying the choroid plexus enter the choroidal fissure adjacent to the lateral geniculate body. The foramen of Monro is the dilated anterior superior limit of the fissure. The choroid plexus is attached to the lips of the fissure by the taeniae thalami and fornices.

Lateral mesencephalic sulcus

At this sulcus, cranial nerve IV disappears inferior to the tentorial edge. It is considered a 'safe-entry' point to the midbrain.

Limen insulae

The limen insulae forms the junction point between the anterior and posterior stem of the Sylvian fissure. It is the most lateral limit of the anterior perforated substance and the starting point of the insular cortex. It has a close relationship to the middle cerebral artery (MCA) and branches.

White matter tracts

Knowledge of the functional anatomy of white matter tracts is important. These tracts are taken into consideration in planning surgical trajectories, neurophysiological monitoring and prediction of resulting deficits and strategies for their avoidance. Although deficits from cortical injury potentially may recover due to plasticity, those resulting from disruption of white matter tracts are likely to be permanent. You should be able to establish their virtual anatomical location on standard imaging and have the knowledge regarding imaging techniques such as diffusion tensor imaging (DTI), especially the technical principles and pitfalls and limitations of the studies. The implication of your knowledge on white matter and tracts anatomy will be demonstrated in the discussion of low-grade glioma surgery including imaging, techniques of white matter neurophysiological monitoring and performance of maximum safe resections. In fact, this applies to surgery for many intrinsic lesions such as epilepsy surgery, deep cavernomas and arteriovenous malformations (AVMs). Discussion regarding approaches to intraventricular lesions should include the implication of transgressing these tracts and describing trajectories aiming to minimize the risks.

The arrangements of the white matter fibres are shown in Table 3.1. There are particular anatomical arrangements that are relevant especially for low-grade glioma surgery such as the insula and its deep layers, the sagittal stratum and the temporal stem. Cases discussed in operative Viva may include locations such as the insula, paralimbic or SMA locations. In particular, the arrangements providing language function will be briefly described. There are two systems the dorsal (sensory and motor integration for speech production in dominant hemisphere) and ventral

Table 3.1 Arrangements of white matter tracts

	Hemisphere	Corona radiata	
Projection	Insular region	Internal capsule	
Association	Short	U-fibres	
	Long	Hemisphere Insular region	SLF Arcuate IFOF Optic radiation Cingulum ILF Fornix Extreme capsule Uncinate
Commissural	Corpus callosum Anterior commissure Hippocampal		

IFOF = (inferior) fronto-occipital fasciculus, ILF = inferior longitudinal fasciculus, SLF = superior longitudinal fasciculus.

(language comprehension). The motor output starts in the inferior frontal lobe deep to the operculum and connected to the posterior superior temporal region via the arcuate fasciculus with further connections to the inferior parietal lobule. The arcuate fasciculus is adjacent to the superior longitudinal fasciculus (SLF) and superior to the superior limiting sulcus of the insula. Disruption is manifested as the disconnection type of dysphasia. The inferior fronto-occipital fasciculus (IFOF) (in fact in the absence of a superior equivalent tract it should be labelled as FOF) connects the occipital lobe and association areas to the frontal lobe. White matter fibre dissections can trace it covering the lateral surface of the atrium of the lateral ventricle and may be separated from the fibres of the optic radiation and pass anteriorly deep and superior to the inferior limiting sulcus of the insula to intermingle with the external capsule. Its disruption results in semantic paraphasias. Its identification by awake neurophysiological monitoring would avoid its disruption and would limit the deep resection. Deeper to this layer, possible injury to the fibres of the internal capsule and its blood supply by the perforators through the anterior perforating substance occurs. The uncinate fasciculus connects the deeper orbital frontal region to the anterior temporal. Disruption of this delays generation of speech but mostly recovers unless other tracts such as the inferior longitudinal fasciculus (ILF) are malfunctioning as well. The ILF passes deep to the fusiform gyrus and, in addition, is involved in facial recognition.

The SLF connects the frontal, temporal and parietal lobes. The subcortical white matter network allows complex dynamic brain function processing for language, motor and cognitive functions. The components SLF I, II and III are organized anteroposteriorly with the different components varying in their extension and location within the hemisphere with an additional SLF parieto-temporal connection.

The optic radiation arises at the lateral geniculate body (with possible significant contribution from the pulvinar) of the thalamus and travels initially anteriorly adjacent to the roof of the temporal horn reaching the temporal stem as Myer's loop. It covers the whole lateral aspect of the atrium, being denser inferiorly and lateral approaches to the lateral ventricle would result in visual field deficits of varying degrees.

The cingulum being part of the circuit of Papez is deep to the cingulate sulcus and inferior to the SMA and if disrupted (as the case for surgery in low-grade gliomas adjacent to the SMA) results in additional neurocognitive and behavioural deficits. The Aslant tract connects to the caudate.

White matter tracts

Lateral hemisphere/Sagittal stratum

- SLF/Arcuate fasciculus
  - Superior longitudinal I, II and III, arcuate
  - Vertical occipital
  - Middle longitudinal
- (Inferior) fronto-occipital (IFOF)
- Optic radiation
- Internal capsule, corona radiata
- Tapetum

Others

- Inferior longitudinal (ILF)
- Cingulum
- Corpus callosum

Deep layers of the insula

- Insula
- Extreme capsule
- Claustrum
- External capsule
- Putamen
- GP
- Internal capsule

Operative surgery and surgical anatomy

Introduction to operative surgery

1. Obtain informed consent from the patient, explaining the benefits and risks of the surgical procedure.
2. Ensure the appropriate side is marked.
3. Ensure radiological imaging and equipment is checked.
4. Follow the WHO Surgical Checklist.
5. Note that the procedure will be performed with the patient under general anaesthetic, with a urinary catheter in place and pre-operative antibiotics and steroids provided at the time of induction (if appropriate).
6. Note positioning of the patient.
7. Ensure standard preparation and drape.

As image guidance surgery becomes the standard of care in neurosurgery, it is imperative that surgeons become skilled in the use of neuro-navigational systems. Be familiar with the basic principles of these machines and the use of additional functional imaging modalities such as PET, SPECT, DTI (for fibre tracking) and fMRI scans.

Case 1

A 35-year-old man presents with a World Federation of Neurological Societies (WFNS) grade II subarachnoid haemorrhage (SAH) secondary to anterior circulation aneurysm. His aneurysm is not suitable for endovascular coiling. He has been scheduled for surgery. Please describe your approach for pterional craniotomy.

Pterional craniotomy

- The patient is placed in the supine position with the head elevated and rotated away from the operative side (ensuring the malar eminence is the highest point in the surgical field).
- A pterional incision begins superiorly on the midline at the anterior edge of the hairline (e.g. at the widow's peak) and extended inferiorly (remaining behind the

hairline) to within 1 cm of the superior aspect of the zygoma, 1 cm anterior to the external auditory canal.
- A myocutaneous flap is reflected in one layer.
- A burr hole is placed in the keyhole position while ensuring the orbit is protected.
- Another burr hole is placed just above the zygoma.
- A free bone flap is fashioned.
- The inner table of the frontal bone and greater and lesser wings of the sphenoid are drilled until flush with the anterior cranial fossa floor.
- Dura is opened in a semicircular fashion.
- A brain spatula is used to retract the frontal lobe and to release CSF from the opticocarotid cistern, carefully opening arachnoid membranes.
- Further steps would be to describe careful dissection around the aneurysm and placement of the clip without obstructing the distal vessels.

Case 2

A 22-year-old man presents with headaches and blurred vision. His magnetic resonance imaging (MRI) scan demonstrates a colloid cyst in the anterior third ventricle. He has been scheduled for surgery. Please describe a transcallosal approach. (There may be some preliminary discussion about emergently treating hydrocephalus and the relative merits of endoscopic vs. open surgery [e.g. transcallosal vs. transcortical approaches]).

Transcallosal approach
- The patient is in a supine position with the head in a neutral position (Mayfield three-point pin fixation).
- The head is elevated to 30°.
- A curved skin incision is made over the coronal suture.
  - Approximately, two-thirds anterior and one-third posterior to the coronal suture.
- Two burr holes are placed on the SSS.
- Free bone flap is fashioned with 1 cm on the left and 3 cm on the right side. The craniotomy is about 6 cm in length and 5 cm in width.
- Budde halo retractor system is assembled.
- A U-shaped dural flap is made. A curved durotomy is made with the base over the SSS. The dural edge is then secured and hitched.
- Arachnoid granulation is dissected free from the base.
- Care is taken not to sacrifice the cortical veins.
- Using a hand-held retractor, gentle retraction is placed along the interhemispheric fissure.
- Identify the following structures:
  - Callasomarginal and pericallosal arteries.
  - Cingulate gyrus.
  - Pericallosal arteries.
  - Corpus callosum (pearly white colour).
- When both pericallosal arteries are identified, the callosal section of <2 cm is made between the two arteries (avoid the penetrating branches).
- The cauterized ependymal layer is opened for entry into the lateral ventricles.

- The orientation of the ventricle is confirmed by the configuration of the choroid plexus and thalamostriate vein, which courses anteriorly in a medial direction to reach the foramen of Monro.
- Foraminal entry via the foramen of Monro, especially if it has been dilated by the presence of hydrocephalus, is the least traumatic. The choroidal fissure can be opened posteriorly to enlarge the foramen of Monro.
- Lateral retraction at this point within the ventricle may damage the genu of the corpus callosum.
- If the lesion is not accessible via foraminal entry, the interforniceal approach is utilized. The interforniceal approach is achieved by a callosotomy that is as close as possible to the midline.
- A colloid cyst wall is firm, smooth and greyish in colour. Attachment of cyst at tela choroidae is identified and released.

Transcallosal resection of a colloid cyst

Key points and safety considerations

- Position head and location of craniotomy – note location of burr holes.
- Avoid compression of SSS by medial retractor (if used).
- Take care to avoid damage of supplementary motor cortex (by retraction) or cingulate gyrus (by misidentifying the callosomarginal artery as pericallosal artery).
- Perform septum pellucidotomy.
- Take care in avoiding damage to the fornix.
- Insert an EVD for safety to prevent post-operative hydrocephalus from intraventricular haemorrhage.

Potential pitfalls

Anatomical landmarks – do not rely on image guidance alone because the coronal suture is in line with the foramen of Monro in the true coronal plane.

If a cyst is located in the posterior third ventricular roof, it is better to choose a subforniceal transchoroidal approach via taenia fornices rather than divide the fornix.

Identify the correct foramen of Monro (lateralization).

Case 3

A 57-year-old woman presents with headaches, facial pain and an unsteady gait. Her MRI scan demonstrates a petroclival tumour. She has been scheduled for surgery. Clearly, this is a difficult operation, and it should be acknowledged as such by the candidate.

Subtemporal transtentorial approach

- The patient is placed in a lateral position.
- The head is elevated to 30°.
- Skin incision: A reverse horseshoe skin incision is made starting from the zygoma 1 cm anterior to the tragus, extending above the pinna and curving down about 2 cm behind the mastoid.

- The scalp flap is reflected inferiorly down the zygoma. Care is taken not to enter the external auditory canal.
- A burr hole is made in the squamous portion of the temporal bone immediately above the roof of the zygoma.
- A temporal craniotomy is made with its posterior extent just above the mastoid, and additional bone is removed down to the middle fossa floor.
- Mastoid air cells are waxed.
- Extradural dissection is performed from a lateral-to-medial and posterior-to-anterior direction to avoid stretching the greater superficial petrosal nerve (GSPN) branch of the facial nerve.
- The following landmarks are identified: Tegmen tympani, arcuate eminence, lesser superficial petrosal nerve (LSPN), GSPN, middle meningeal artery and mandibular branch of the trigeminal nerve. The LSPN can be distinguished from the GSPN by its joining with the middle meningeal artery at the foramen spinosum.
- The dura is opened with a T-shaped incision along the inferior temporal lobe and with a vertical limb along the middle fossa floor.
- Retraction of the temporal lobe is performed with the aid the microscope.
- Temporal lobe elevation is limited by vein of Labbé.
- Cranial nerve IV is identified; the division of the tentorium begins immediately posterior, near the petrous ridge. The tentorial division is extended 3–4 cm posterolaterally and a couple of millimetres posterior to the superior petrosal sinus without injuring the sigmoid sinus. The division of the tentorium is carried in an anterolateral direction into the middle fossa and across the superior petrosal sinus with ligatures or clips. This results in a triangular flap with a view down onto the clivus.

Subtemporal approach

Key points and safety considerations

- Consider a lumbar drain (if no contraindication, e.g. a large mass). CSF retrieval from cisterns may require retraction.
- Preserve vein of Labbé.
- Be aware of the location of cranial nerve IV at tentorial hiatus.
- In true petro-clival meningiomas, the VI cranial nerve is the most vulnerable to injury.

Potential pitfalls

Anatomy of vein of Labbé and variations in number and configuration.

Case 4

A 63-year-old woman presents with progressive visual loss and ophthalmoplegia. Her MRI scan demonstrates a pituitary macroadeoma. Her pituitary function tests (including prolactin) are normal. She has been scheduled for surgery. Generally speaking, the endoscopic approach is now more frequently employed than microscopic, but one should be prepared to talk through the principles of both techniques.

Endoscopic endonasal transsphenoidal approach

This is a bi-nostril four-hand technique. Ideally, an operation performed together by neurosurgeons and ENT surgeons.

- The patient is placed in a supine position with the head resting on a donut.
- Nasal decongestants.
- In complicated or recurrent cases, the aide of neuronavigation such as the AXIEM system may be considered.

Relevant surgical anatomy

- The bony nasal septum is formed by the perpendicular plate of the ethmoid and vomer bone. It is attached to the rostrum of the sphenoid sinus (SS) in the midline, frequently deviated to one side. If prominent and angulated deviation is present, it is called a 'septal spur'; then, this may compromise access and needs correction.
- On the lateral wall of the nasal cavity, the superior and middle turbinates are parts of the ethmoid bone, while the inferior turbinate is a separate bone. The SS communicates with the nasal cavity via the sphenoid osteum located in the naso-ethmoidal recess superior and medial to the superior turbinate.
- The paraclival ICA, on either side of the clivus as visible through the SS, is the vertical petrous or lacerum segment of the intracavernous internal carotid artery (ICA). The parasellar ICA is the carotid syphon of the intracavernous ICA.
- The lateral opticocarotid recess (OCR), which is between the parasellar ICA (carotid canal) and the impression of the II nerve, marks the strut of the anterior clinoid process (optic strut) and can be well aerated. The medial OCR is located above the level of the middle clinoid process and marks the medial CS compartment and acts as the gateway landmark to extended transplanum endoscopic approaches.
- The posterior septal branch of the sphenopalatine artery as it emerges in the middle meatus. This provides the blood supply to the pedicle of the nasoseptal flap harvested over the nasal septum. It passes inferior to the sphenoid ostium, and care should be exerted to preserve it by widening the ostea to access the SS.

Endonasal endoscopic access

- On entry to the nasal cavity with 0 degree scope, the anatomical landmarks are inspected and the middle turbinate of followed and eventually the sphenoid osteum is located.
- Depending on preference, the inferior prominence of the middle turbinate is either excised or mobilized laterally to allow a space to place the scope during the procedure. In doing so, care must be taken to avoid pushing the turbinate laterally by placing the instrument superiorly as the attachment of the turbinate to the cribriform plate may result in a fracture and a resulting CSF leak from this area which can be difficult to repair. The middle turbinate sometimes harbours an air cell – 'concha bulosa' and is very bulky and needs a reduction to provide space.
- If the sphenoid osteum is covered by mucosa and initially not visible, it can be located by reference to its relationship to the choana (connection of nasal cavity

to nasopharynx). It is about 15 mm superior to the choana in the naso-ethmoidal recess (using a known 3-mm-wide dissector and moving it 4 or 5 times upward from the choana and gently advancing it through the mucosa would help to locate the osteum.

- The SS is then widely opened by removing its anterior wall and performing a posterior septostomy.
- The SS contains several bony septae; some of these are attached to the carotid canal. Clearance of this septae provides a wide SS cavity for the procedure. Posteriorly near attachments in vicinity to the carotid canal, these are flattened with. Drill rather than fracturing by using a rongeur is advised to avoid carotid injury.
- The sella floor is identified (beware of the presellar and cochal variations of the SS) and is thinned with a drill and removed to expose the dura with the extreme extensions being the blue colouration of the CS on either side and the superior and inferior inter-cavernous sinuses.
- A cruciate X-shaped opening of the dura is made with care not to cause excessive bleeding from extension into the venous sinuses. Beware that the bone may be dehiscent over the carotid canal.
- For macroadenomas (which is the case here) that are invariably soft in consistency the use of curretes and suction starting by clearing the inferior and lateral aspects of the sella first, and eventually, the diaphragma will descent indicating adequate decompression.
- A 30 degree scope can be used to inspect for any residual tumour.
- Try to preserve the gland that is usually compressed against the dural wall and identified by its colour and firmer consistency. The side of deviation of the stalk on the pre-operative MRI may help in predicting its location.
- For microadenomas (not this case), identification of the tumour depends upon its different colour and softer consistency. To achieve cure in secretory microadenomas, wider resection may be required as it is possible that the tumour extends beyond the margins of the pseudocapsule.
- CSF leak repair is performed by applying a fat graft from the subcutaneous tissue of the thigh or abdominal wall. If more extensive a nasoseptal flap is applied, it ensures no kinking of the vascular pedicle and good contact with the surrounding skull base bone.

Transsphenoidal approach – Microscopic

- The patient is placed in a supine position with the head in a neutral position resting on a donut.
- Equipment: Image intensifier and a microscope are both in place.
- The lateral thigh is prepared.
- 0.25% xylocaine and adrenaline infiltrated into the nasal mucosa.
- Otrivine nasal spray is used to reduce nasal congestion.
- Apply adequate aqueous-based antiseptic solution.
- The operative surgeon stands at the cranial end of the operative table or on the right side of the patient.
- Right-sided transnasal paraseptal approach is used.
- A curved incision is made along the mucocutaneous junction along the columella or deep over the bony/cartilaginous junction of the nasal septum, e.g. Kellihan.

- Sub-perichondral dissection is performed.
- A long hand-held nasal speculum (e.g. Kellihan) is used to advance and fracture the perpendicular plate of the ethmoid bone.
- Orientation along the sagittal plane is checked regularly with fluoroscopy.
- Identify the sphenoid ostium and keel of the rostrum.
- Anterior wall of SS is entered using an osteotome or drill.
- The opening may be widened with Kerrison rongeurs.
- Septation within the SS is identified on a CT scan.
- Cruciate durotomy is made.
- Use angled ring curettes, tumour forceps and suction to gently debulk the tumour.
- Apply a Valsalva manoeuvre to deliver the remaining tumour.

Complications of the transsphenoidal approach

- Epistaxis.
- Nasal perforation.
- Sinusitis.
- Visual impairment (ophthalmoplegia and loss of vision).
- Transient/permanent diabetes insipidus.
- CSF rhinorrhoea.
- Meningitis.
- Damage to surrounding structures (cavernous sinus, intracavernous cranial nerves and carotid artery).

Transsphenoidal resection of pituitary adenoma

Key points and safety considerations

Consider image guidance in cases that are revision, extended approaches or have challenging sellar anatomy when performing endoscopic or microscopic-assisted transsphenoidal surgery.

Avoid carotid injury – identify the 'kissing' carotids, avoid avulsion of a laterally placed intrasphenoid sinus septum inserting into the carotid canal and carefully identify anatomical landmarks and midline when drilling.

The order of resection of large macroadenomas is to avoid premature descent of the diaphragm sellae.

For endoscopic cases, different angled scopes are used to inspect the sella for complete surgical resection.

Potential pitfalls

Be aware of the true invasion of cavernous sinus vs. compression.
Be aware of the need for total resection for secretory vs. nonsecretory adenomas.

Case 5

A 24-year-old man presents with headache, visual deterioration and vomiting. His MRI scan demonstrated non-communicating (obstructive) hydrocephalus secondary to aqueductal stenosis. He has been scheduled for surgery.

Endoscopic third ventriculostomy

- The patient is placed in a supine position with the patient's head in a neutral position on a horseshoe headrest.
- The head is then elevated to minimize excessive CSF loss and air entry.
- A linear, S- or U-curved-shaped skin incision is made.
- A burr hole is placed 3 cm lateral to the midline and 1 cm anterior to the coronal suture.
- A cruciate durotomy is made.
- No. 14 French peel-away catheter is then used to cannulate the lateral ventricle.
- The stylet is removed to ensure its placement into the ventricular system.
- The two leaves are peeled away and stapled to the drapes.
- A rigid endoscope is passed through the sheath and the lateral ventricle is visualized.
- Important structures to identify are foramen of Monro, choroid plexus and thamalostriate veins.
- The scope is advanced further through the foramen into the third ventricle. Be careful not to traumatize the fornix.
- The landmarks located on the floor of the third ventricle are the following:
  - Mammillary bodies posteriorly.
  - Infundibular recess anteriorly.
  - Thin, transparent floor of the third ventricle.
  - Basilar artery visualized through the thinned floor.
- French Fogarty balloon catheter is advanced through the opening into the floor, 0.2 mL of fluid is instilled into the balloon, and the balloon is inflated to widen the newly created aperture.
- After advancing the endoscope into the prepontine cistern, the arachnoid bands are released.
- Inspect for CSF flow through the fenestration.
- Consider insertion of a ventricular access device or an external ventricular drain if the patient was previously shunt dependent, symptomatic pre-operatively, or if the procedure was complicated by intraoperative bleeding.

Endoscopic third ventriculostomy (ETV)

Key points and safety considerations

Position of burr hole and trajectory.
Anatomical landmarks.
Location and performance of stoma to avoid stretching or damage of basilar artery or P1 perforators.
Anatomical attachment of second membrane/medial extension of Lilliquist's membrane.

Potential pitfalls

Do not proceed without adequate visualization of anatomical landmarks.
Ensure adequate stoma and opening of all membranes.

= Age Score + Etiology Score + Previous Shunt Score
≈ percentage probability of ETV success

SCORE	AGE +	ETIOLOGY +	PREVIOUS SHUNT
0	<1 MONTH	POST-INFECTIOUS	PREVIOUS SHUNT
10	<1 MONTH TO <6 MONTHS		NO PREVIOUS SHUNT
20		MYELOMENINGOCELE INTRA-VENTRICULAR HEMORRHAGE NON-TECTAL BRAIN TUMOUR	
30	6 MONTHS TO <1 YEAR	AQUEDUCTAL STENOSIS TECTAL TUMOUR OTHER ETIOLOGY	
40	1 YEAR TO <10 YEARS		

Figure 3.1 The ETV success score (ETVSS).

- If an endoscopic biopsy of an intracranial lesion is also required, perform ETV first because bleeding from the biopsy site may obscure the view and preclude completion of the ETV.
- The ETV success score is designed to predict the results (Figure 3.1).
- The total is the % of the predicted success rate.

Case 6

A 32-year-old woman presents with a chronic history of neck pain and intermittent suboccipital headaches that are worse with neck extension and coughing. Her MRI scan demonstrated a Chiari malformation type I with no evidence of hydrocephalus. She has been scheduled for surgery.

Foramen magnum decompression

- Procedure is performed in a prone position with the head secured on Mayfield three-point pin skull clamp.
- The patient's neck is placed in a 'military tuck position' (neck extended and flexed at the atlanto-occipital junction).
- Ensure no venous congestion.
- Linear midline incision is made extending from the level of inion (external occipital protuberance) to the C2 spinous process.
- Bilateral paraspinous muscles are stripped with monopolar diathermy.
- Subperiosteal dissection over C1, C2 and occiput is performed.
- Identify the C2 spinous process and the inion.

- Four burr holes are made and connected by using a craniotome. The bone flap is then elevated.
- The posterior arch of C1 may need to be removed.
- Ensure adequate haematosis.
- Careful Y-shaped durotomy is made while keeping the arachnoid layer intact.

Foramen magnum decompression

Key points and safety considerations

Ensure correct indications for surgery, differentiate between those with or without syrinx and look for significant anterior additional pathology.

If hydrocephalus is present, best to insert a shunt first.

Avoid overflexion while positioning (± somatosensory evoked potentials [SSEPs]).

Tailor bone decompression.

Protect tonsillar loops of posterior inferior cerebellar artery (PICA).

Consider checking CSF flow at the end of the procedure with ultrasound guidance.

Potential pitfalls

Describe the same procedure regardless of presentation and anatomical variation.

Be able to debate reasons for the chosen technique (e.g. opening dura ± opening arachnoid).

Case 7

A 54-year-old man presents with craniocervical pain associated with numbness and tingling of the fingers. On clinical examination, there was evidence of long tract signs (spasticity, hyperreflexia). His MRI scan demonstrated intradural foramen magnum tumour. He has been scheduled for surgery.

Far lateral approach to the skull base

- The patient is placed in a park bench position with the head secured on Mayfield three-point pin skull clamp.
- Check the following
  - Ensure no venous congestion.
  - The pressure areas are protected.
  - Equipment, radiological imaging and microscope are checked pre-operatively.
- A retromastoid 'inverted hockey stick' incision is performed with the lateral limb extending below the mastoid process and the medial limb just below C3, if the lesion is below the foramen magnum.
  - Identify the superior nuchal line and follow the midline (C3 level).
- Sub-periosteal dissection of the paraspinous muscles is performed down to the level C2 and C3 spinous processes.
- Occipital bone is exposed.
- Myocutaneous flap is created and retracted infero-laterally.
- Lateral mass of C1 and vertebral artery are exposed. Vertebral artery is identified entering the dura just above C1 arch at the vertebral notch.

- Venous bleeding is controlled with diathermy.
- Depending on the size, position and type of lesion, the suboccipital craniotomy is extended to include the lateral condyle and rim of foramen magnum.
- The dura is opened in a curvilinear fashion or with three lateral triangular leaves based on the transverse sinus, sigmoid sinus and vertebral artery.

Case 8

A 45-year-old woman presents with unilateral hearing loss, tinnitus and unsteady gait. Her MRI scan demonstrated a vestibular schwannoma centred on the internal acoustic meatus (IAM). She has been scheduled for surgery.

Retrosigmoid approach

- The patient is placed in the park bench position.
- Ensure
  - No venous congestion.
  - Facial nerve monitoring application.
  - Insertion of a lumbar drain (ensure absence of large mass or obstructive hydrocephalus) and urinary catheter.
  - Pressure areas are protected.
- Bony landmarks – Mastoid process and external occipital protuberance are identified.
- Pathway of transverse sinus is identified.
- A postauricular curvilinear incision is made 2 cm behind the mastoid tip extending the cephalad above the transverse sinus and caudal to include the mastoid tip.
- The muscles are reflected away by the use of diathermy. A cuff of periosteum is maintained to assist with dual closure at the end of the operation.
- Check the landmarks: asterion and mastoid.
- A burr hole is made at the asterion.
- A craniectomy is performed until both sigmoid sinus and transverse sinus are visible and inferiorly until the foramen magnum is palpable.
- Exposed mastoid air cells are occluded with bone wax.
- If there is bleeding from the mastoid emissary vein entering the transverse and sigmoid sinus, this may be controlled with Gelfoam and patties.
- Budde halo retractor is assembled.
- Cruciate durotomy is performed at the junction of the transverse and sigmoid sinus.
- The cerebellum is relaxed by releasing CSF from the arachnoid.
- A narrow 3-mm brain spatula is introduced parallel and below the superior petrosal.

Retrosigmoid craniotomy

Key points and safety considerations

Landmarks of transverse and sigmoid sinuses – mastoid and digastric groove.

CSF retrieval from the cisterna magna.

Avoidance of excessive cerebellar retraction.

Correct identification of cranial nerves – landmarks.

Potential pitfalls

Discussion of retrosigmoid versus translabyrinthine approaches.

Knowledge of neurophysiological cranial nerve monitoring.

'Pros and cons' of preservation of vein of Dandy.

Case 9

A 66-year-old man presents with progressive bilateral hand weakness, in that he is now dropping objects. His cervical MRI scan demonstrated cervical spondylosis with spinal cord compression. He has been scheduled for surgery.

Anterior cervical discectomy and fusion

- The patient is placed in a supine position with the neck slightly extended.
- A right-sided approach is used. The examiner may ask you why and the potential differences in complications vs. a left-sided approach. Know the course of the recurrent laryngeal nerve, thoracic duct, the sympathetic chain, etc.
- Linear skin incision is made along Langer's line at the correct level. The examiner may ask you about these landmarks.
- Exposure is performed in layers.
- Platysma is cut and undermined.
- The investing layer of cervical fascia is divided along the anterior border of sternocleidomastoid (SCM) to define the plane between the carotid sheath laterally and the larynx, trachea and oesophagus medially.
- A combination of a careful sharp and blunt dissection is used, initially medial to SCM and lateral to the superior belly of omohyoid.
- At this stage, it is essential to palpate for the carotid artery and continue medially to the carotid artery toward the spine. A handheld Cloward retractor is used.
- Blunt dissection of prevertebral fascia using peanut sponges is used to expose both longus colli muscles.
- The level is confirmed with X-ray. Use a bent spinal needle in the disc space as a marker to identify the correct level.
- Once this is achieved, Cloward's or black-belt retractors are inserted underneath the medial border of both longus colli muscles.
- A box-shaped incision is made over the anterior longitudinal ligament (ALL) and extended laterally to the uncal-vertebral joint. The anterior annulus is incised.
- Using a microscope, the disc fragments are removed using rongeurs and curettes.
- A high-speed drill is used to gently burr the bony end plates and to remove osteophytes and the posterior uncinate process.
- The dissection is continued laterally until the upslope of the uncinate process is encountered.
- Once the posterior osteophyte is removed with a high-speed drill, the posterior longitudinal ligament is removed using a 1-mm Kerrison rongeur.
- Careful exploration with a blunt hook probe alongside the nerve root confirms adequate compression.

- A trial cage is inserted under X-ray guidance.
- The cage (with a bone graft) is gently tapped into the place with a hammer and mallet.
- An anterior cervical plate may be placed at this point.
- Haemostasis is achieved.
- A gravity drain is inserted.

Complications of ACDF

- Infection.
- Bleeding (including haematoma).
- CSF leakage.
- Recurrence.
- Failure.
- Further surgery.
- Progression.
- Paralysis (nerve root or spinal cord injury).
- Hoarse voice (recurrent laryngeal injury).
  - It is common to ask about this potential complication as the potential risk increases with lower levels. If asked to totally avoid this complication (e.g. in professional singers), consider the alternative posterior foraminotomy approach.
- Hypoglossal nerve or superior laryngeal nerve injury.
- Swallowing difficulties.
- Pneumothorax.
- Oesophageal perforation.
- Carotid artery injury.
- Horner's syndrome.
- Pseudoarthrosis.
- Instability.
- Instrumentation failure.

Case 10

A 33-year-old man presents with back pain coupled with right leg pain radiating into his sole, coupled with a foot drop. His lumbar MRI scan demonstrated a large right-sided L4/5 lumbar disc protrusion. He has been scheduled for surgery.

Lumbar microdiscectomy

- The patient is placed in a prone position on a Wilson frame or Montreal mattress.
- Pre-operative X-ray is used to confirm the correct level.
- Surgery is conducted from the ipsilateral to the symptomatic side.
- A midline linear skin incision is performed.
- Exposure is performed in layers.
- Subperiosteal paraspinous muscle dissection is achieved with monopolar diathermy.
- The interspace is identified.
- A foraminotomy is performed using a mixture of Kerrison punches and rongeurs.

- Medial aspect of the facet is removed.
- The bone edges are waxed to achieve haemostasis.
- With the assistance of the operative microscope, ligamentum flavum is excised using sharp and blunt dissection. Bipolar coagulation of epidural veins may be required.
- The nerve root is identified and then gently retracted/protected medially.
- If a free disc fragment is seen in the canal, it is removed with a pituitary rongeur.
- If the fragment is under the thecal sac, the fragment can be brought forward with a nerve hook.
- If the disc fragment is contained within the annulus, a further incision (rectangle or a single cut parallel to the nerve root) is made over the annulus.
- If the disc fragment is intradural, the dura will need to be opened.

Complications of lumbar microdiscectomy

- Infection.
- Bleeding (including haematoma).
- CSF leakage.
- Recurrence.
- Further surgery.
- Progression.
- Paralysis (nerve root or cauda equina injury).
- Sphincter dysfunction (bowel, urinary or sexual).
- Instability.
- Rarely, internal iliac vessels injury, especially at the L4/L5 level.

Overall outcome

- 70–75% of patients experience a significant improvement in their leg pain.
- 20–25% of patients improve but report persistent leg pain.
- 5% of patients have no benefit at all.
- 1% of patients deteriorate (leg pain).

Special case: Far lateral discectomy for extraforaminal disc herniation

- The patient is placed in a prone position on a Wilson frame or Montreal mattress.
- Pre-operative X-ray is used to confirm needle placement on the correct level.
- Surgery is conducted from the ipsilateral symptomatic side.
- Standard preparation and drape are performed.
- Paramedian intertransverse approach: a linear incision 2.5 cm off the midline is made.
- Paraspinous muscles are split along the line of the fibres to expose the transverse process and facet joint.
- Intraoperative X-ray is used to confirm the correct level.
- The operative microscope is used.
- The intertransverse ligament is incised and reflected.
- Careful dissection is carried out to expose the pedicle and pars interarticularis to identify the roof of the foramen.
- The exiting nerve root can be seen underneath the pars.
- The root is then mobilized caudally to expose the prolapsed disc.

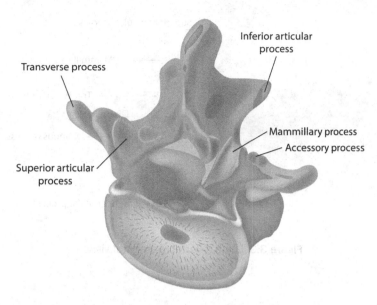

Inferior articular process

Transverse process

Mammillary process

Accessory process

Superior articular process

Figure 3.2 Lumbar vertebra.

Case 11

A 52-year-old female presents with low back pain and bilateral leg pain and paraesthesia. She has an L4/L5 spondylolisthesis with pars defect.

Lumbar pedicle screw fixation

- Pre-operative planning (X-rays, CT scan and MRI scan) for deciding the bone quality, pedicle transverse diameter and screw trajectory may be required. The advantages and disadvantages of free hand, X-ray guided and 3D navigation may be discussed.
- The patient is placed in the prone position on a Wilson frame or Montreal mattress.
- Pre-operative X-ray is used to confirm the correct level.
- Midline linear skin incision is performed. Exposure is performed in layers.
- Monopolar cautery is done through fascia in midline to the spinous processes.
- Bilateral subperiosteal dissection of paraspinal muscles exposes the transverse processes.
- Self-retaining retractors are inserted (Figures 3.2 and 3.3).

Entry point for lumbar pedicle screw

An entry point is the junction of the lateral facet and the transverse process or bisection of a vertical line through the facet joints and a horizontal line through the transverse process. The key anatomical points are the facet joint, transverse process and pars interarticularis (Figures 3.4 and 3.5).

- After decorticating the pedicle entry site with a burr and penetrating the site with an awl, a curved or straight pedicle probe is used to develop a path for the screw through the cancellous bone of the pedicle into the vertebral body.
- The coronal plane angle increases approximately 5° per level from L1 to sacrum.

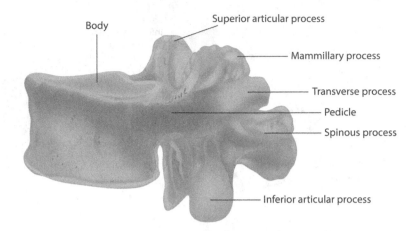

Figure 3.3 Lumbar vertebra, sagittal view.

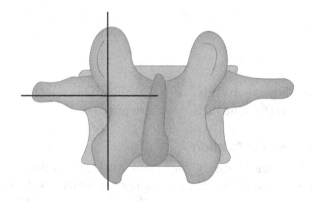

Figure 3.4 Lumbar pedicle entry point.

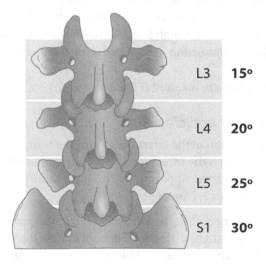

Figure 3.5 Coronal lumbar spine.

- A pedicle feeler is inserted down the created pathway to confirm the pedicle walls are intact.
- The pedicles are then tapped.
- After cannulation and confirmation of the pedicle with the appropriate trajectory, the largest possible pedicle screw is placed (length: determined by measuring the length of the probe from the pedicle entry site to a depth of 50–80% of the vertebral body).
- The screws usually have a diameter of 4.5–7 mm, and a length of 35–50 mm.
- After pedicle screw placement, the transverse process and the lateral aspects of the facet joints are decorticated, the pedicle screws are connected to a rod and top locking set screws are applied.
- Bone graft is then applied along the decorticated transverse processes.

Case 12

A 31-year-old man was involved in a motorbike accident. He was thrown off his motorbike when he was hit by a moving vehicle. He presents with severe back pain. He is neurologically intact. His lumbar CT scan demonstrates an unstable Chance fracture of the L1 vertebrae. He has been scheduled for minimally invasive surgery.

MIS pedicle screw fixation

- There should be pre-operative consideration as the length of the construct (often two up and two down for a unstable fracture), the likely length and diameter of screws at each level should be written on a whiteboard, care and attention around other injuries (especially chest).
- Due care is taken to place the patient prone on a Jackson table with several people to assist in log rolling the patient (formal log roll).
- One needs to ensure that there is adequate room for the C-arm (or O-arm) navigation to rotate around the patient without the pillar of the table, or anaesthetic tubing, getting in the way.
- At each level, one must position the C-arm such that on AP, the end plates are horizontal and spinous processes are central. On lateral, one should also ensure that the X-ray is a 'true' lateral.
- The Jamshedi needle should enter pedicle at the two o'clock and ten o'clock positions.
- A stab incision is made just lateral to this point. The Jamshedi is docked on the bone and a mark is made on the needle 2 cm from the skin. The needle should not breach the medial pedicle until the mark is reached.
- AP and lateral X-rays are used to safely advance the needle.
- Once within a vertebral body, the stylet is removed and replaced with a guidewire. The needle is removed leaving the guidewire in situ.
- A cannulated tap is placed over the guidewire.
- A cannulated screw is then placed on the guidewire and advanced to the position being careful not to advance the guidewire.
- Once all screws have been placed, the rods are placed subcutaneously into the screw heads.
- Set screws are locked.

Case 13

A 74-year-old man presents with impaired memory, gait disturbance and urinary incontinence. His MRI scan demonstrated communicating hydrocephalus. He will undergo lumbar infusion to investigate normal pressure hydrocephalus.

Lumbar infusion studies

- Pressure recording was calibrated stepwise between 0 and 50 mmHg.
- The initial steady-state CSF pressure was recorded (until a stable initial pressure curve for at least 10 min was obtained) before starting a constant rate (0.80 mL/min) infusion of Ringer's solution.
- The CSF pressure is continuously recorded through the other needle via the pressure-monitoring device connected to a printer.
- The CSF pressure is recorded continuously during a period of at least 45 minutes to establish a steady-state pressure plateau representing the pressure level at which absorption balanced infusion.
- If steady-state plateau pressure exceeds 22 mmHg, intervention (shunt insertion) is likely to be beneficial.

Case 14

An 83-year-old woman presents with severe stabbing electric facial pain in a V1 and V2 disturbance. Her MRI scan demonstrated vascular compression of the trigeminal nerve at the root entry zone. She has been scheduled for surgery (see Table 3.2). Explain the results and outcomes for each operative approach.

Percutaneous trigeminal rhizotomy (PTR)

This is a glycerol technique. Other options include balloon compression or radiofrequency lesioning. One should be prepared to talk about at least one of these techniques.

Table 3.2 Results of surgical treatments for trigeminal neuralgia

	Radiofrequency rhizotomy	Balloon compression	Glycerol injection	Microvascular decompression
Total number of patients treated	500	759	1217	1417
Initial pain relief	98%	93%	91%	98%
Recurrence rate	20%	21%	54%	15%
Facial numbness	98%	72%	60%	2%
Anaesthesia dolorosa	0.2%	0.1%	1.8%	0%
Corneal anaesthesia	3%	1.5%	3.7%	0.05%
Perioperative morbidity	0.6%	17%	1%	10%

Source: Adapted from Taha JM, Tew JM. Comparison of surgical treatments for trigeminal neuralgia: reevaluation of radiofrequency rhizotomy. Neurosurgery 1996; 38(5): 865–71.)

- Symptomatic side is marked.
- The patient is placed supine in a neutral position.
- Hartel's anatomical landmark is used to guide the needle with the aid of fluoroscopy.

Three anatomical landmarks are identified on the patient's face:

1. The point supero-lateral to the zygoma and 3 cm in front of the tragus.
2. The point at the intersection of the same axial plane and the midpupillary line.
3. The point 3 cm lateral to the mouth's corner on the bicommissural line.
    - 5 mL of xylocaine 1% with adrenaline (epinephrine) is used as local infiltration.
    - Placing your index finger inside the mouth, a 22G spinal needle is used to guide the needle toward the foramen ovale.
    - X-ray guides the needle to the correct location in the trigeminal cistern.
    - The foramen ovale is seen through the pterygomandibular and infratemporal space as an oval structure at the top of the petrous pyramid.
    - The patient may wince when the needle penetrates the foramen.
    - When the tip of the cannula is located inside the arachnoid of a trigeminal cistern, there may be spontaneous egress of CSF.
    - Iohexol is injected into the cistern as the table is tilted upward to outline Meckel's cave.
    - The inferior edge of the Gasserian ganglion can be seen as the superior edge of the outlined space. The amount of iohexol to fill the cistern is measured by injecting it until the dye overflows into the posterior fossa. The iohexol is withdrawn, and anhydrous glycerol is injected into the same area to fill the cistern.

Case 15

A 34-year-old man sustains a severe head injury following a motorcycle crash. His CT scan demonstrated a diffuse SAH and sulci effacement. He has been scheduled for surgery.

Insertion of an Intracranial pressure (ICP) bolt

- The patient is placed supine with the head in a neutral position.
- Kocher's point (coronal) places the catheter in the frontal horn. If no clinical indications, select the non-dominant hemisphere (right side).
- Entry site is 2–3 cm from the midline in the mid-pupillary line and 1 cm anterior to the coronal suture.
- Open the cranial access kit and the ICP bolt in a sterile fashion.
- Stab incision is performed over the planned burr hole site.
- Place a twist drill hole through skull without penetrating the dura.
- Use the safety nut on the drill to prevent plunging.
- Screw the bolt into the skull until finger tight.
- Open the dura with a probe (available in the cranial access kit).
- Direct the catheter perpendicular to the brain's surface to a depth of 5 cm.
- Confirm a waveform is present.
- Tighten the bolt around the catheter to secure in place.

Case 16

A 55-year-old woman presents with a sudden onset of severe headache, vomiting and photophobia. While in the emergency department, she becomes confused and drowsy, and her GCS drops. Her CT scan demonstrated an extensive SAH with intra-ventricular extension. She has been scheduled for surgery.

External ventricular drainage (ventriculostomy)

- The patient is placed supine with the head in a neutral position.
- Kocher's point (coronal) places the catheter in the frontal horn. If no clinical indications, select the non-dominant hemisphere (right side).
- Entry site is 2–3 cm from the midline in the mid-pupillary line and 1 cm anterior to the coronal suture.
- A burr hole is created by holding the perforator perpendicular to the skull.
- Dura is opened.
- Bipolar cautery is used to coagulate the dural edges.
- A ventricular catheter is inserted perpendicular to the brain surface to a depth of 5–6 cm and aimed towards the ipsilateral medial canthus. An antibiotic-impregnated catheter is recommended.
- The stylet is withdrawn from the catheter to check for CSF flow.
- The opening pressure is measured.
- A tunnelling device is attached to the distal end of the catheter. Stabilize the catheter at the burr hole and tunnel the distal portion under the galea aponeurosis to a skin exit site at least 5 cm away from the entry point.
- Reconfirm CSF drainage.
- Close the galea aponeurosis with 2.0 Vicryl and apply skin clips.
- The catheter is secured to the scalp with a U stitch with 3.0 nylon.
- The distal end of the catheter is connected to a drainage system.

Post-operative considerations

- Send CSF for analysis (biochemistry, bacteriology ± cytology).

Case 17

A 28-year-old woman presents with headaches, vomiting and abducens palsy. On fundoscopy, there is evidence of papilloedema. Her CT scan demonstrated hydro-cephalus with periventricular lucency. She has been scheduled for surgery.

Ventriculoperitoneal (VP) shunt insertion

- The patient is placed supine with the head turned 90° to the opposite side with an ipsilateral shoulder roll in place.
- Shunt is assembled.
- If there are no specific clinical indications, select the non-dominant hemisphere (right side) as the entry site. Scalp incision is a small semilunar scalp flap or linear incision.
  - Frontal approach: Kocher's point (coronal) places the catheter in the frontal horn. Entry site: 2–3 cm from the midline in the mid-pupillary line and 1 cm anterior to the coronal suture.

- Occipital–parietal approach: Frazier burr hole: 3–4 cm from the midline, 6–7 cm above the inion.
- Parietal boss: Flat portion of the parietal bone, 3 cm above and 3 cm posterior to the top of the pinna.
- Abdominal approach: Create a horizontal incision, 2 cm lateral and 2 cm superior to the umbilicus. The anterior rectus sheath is incised. Rectus muscle is split in layers. Long clamps are placed on posterior rectus sheath and then incised. Additional clamps are placed on the peritoneum.
- Burr hole
  - Retractors pulled caudally in order for the burr hole to be placed 1 cm below the incision to ensure that no hardware lies under the suture line. The burr hole is created by holding the perforator perpendicular to the skull.
- Dural opening
  - Bipolar cautery is used to coagulate the dural edges.
- Tunnel the shunt from the scalp to the abdominal incision by inserting a metal trocar/passer in which the shunt is then passed.
- Cannulate the ventricles. The ventricular catheter is inserted perpendicular to the brain surface.
  - Frontal approach: The catheter is inserted to a depth of 5–6 cm. Aim towards the ipsilateral medial canthus.
  - Occipital-parietal approach: The catheter is inserted to a depth of 8 cm.
  - The stylet is withdrawn from the catheter to ensure CSF flow and to measure the opening pressure.
- Assemble the shunt.
- Connect the value between proximal and distal catheter. Secure with a silk tie.
- Assess catheter placement.
  - Check for spontaneous CSF flow from the distal end.
  - If there is no spontaneous dripping, CSF can be gently aspirated from the distal catheter with a blunt needle.
  - The shunt value is easily pumped.
- Place peritoneal catheter.
  - The shunt is placed in the perineum with non-tooth forceps.
- Close the wound.
  - Ventricular end: Close galea aponeurosis with 2.0 Vicryl and then apply skin clips.
  - Distal end: Close the peritoneum with 2-0 Ethicon (purse–string suture). Apply interrupted Vicryl sutures to the fascia and subcutaneous tissue, and then apply skin clips.

Post-operative considerations

- Send CSF for analysis (biochemistry, bacteriology ± cytology).
- Perform neurological observations.
- The patient can resume eating when bowel sounds are noted (due to a paralytic ileus).
- Obtain a shunt series (AP and lateral skull, chest/abdominal X-rays).

Additional notes

- A valve is a mechanical device that regulates pressure or restricts flow. A valve typically functions as follows: When the difference between the inlet pressure and the outlet pressure exceeds the opening threshold, the valve opens.
- Designs include the following:
  - Silicone rubber mitre valve.
  - Silicone rubber slit valve.
  - Rubber diaphragm valve.
  - Metallic spring ball valve.
- The opening pressure can be low, medium or high, which corresponds to 5, 10, and 15 mmHg, respectively.
- Anti-siphon device is a mobile membrane that narrows an orifice in response to negative pressure. When a patient stands, there can be a siphon effect.
- Requirements of an ideal shunt are the following:
  - The resistance of an open shunt should be taken together with the natural CSF.
  - Outflow resistance (usually increased in hydrocephalus) should be close to the normal resistance to CSF outflow, e.g. 6–10 mmHg mL^{-1} min^{-1}.
  - Flow should remain constant under constant pressure conditions.
  - Flow through the shunt should not depend on the body posture or be affected by body temperature, external (environmental) pressure (within the physiological range for subcutaneous pressure) or the pulsatile component of CSF pressure.
  - Opening and closing pressures (the pressure at which flow starts and ceases) should remain constant under the conditions listed previously.
- Reversal of flow through the shunt should be impossible.

Discuss the various settings, adjustments, advantages and disadvantages of programmable shunts.

Special cases: Craniotomies to debulk underlying space-occupying lesions (meningiomas)

Case 18

A 45-year-old woman presents with headaches. Her MRI scan demonstrated a homogeneous densely enhancing mass with a broad base of attachment along the dural border with a 'dural tail'. There is evidence of mass effect. She has been scheduled for surgery.

Convexity meningioma

- Pre-operative steroids and antibiotics are given, and a urinary catheter is inserted.
- The patient is placed supine with the head fixed on a Mayfield three-point pin headrest.
- The head is rotated to the contralateral side to allow easy access to the tumour. The head is positioned so the bone flap overlying the tumour is parallel to the floor and elevated approximately 30°.
- When using the image guidance system, the tumour may be identified and marked on the patient's scalp.

Simpson grade	Definition
I	Macroscopically complete tumour resection with removal of affected dura and underlying bone
II	Macroscopically complete tumour resection with coagulation of affected dura only
III	Macroscopically complete tumour resection without removal of affected dura or underlying bone
IV	Subtotal tumour resection
V	Decompression with or without biopsy

Simpson D. The recurrence of intracranial meningiomas after surgical treatment. *J Neurol Neurosurg Psychiatry* 1957;20:22–39

Figure 3.6 Simpson grading system for meningioma according to the extent of resection.

- Preservation of uninvolved cortical veins.
- A curve scalp incision is used based on the location and size of tumour.
- The temporalis muscle is incised and elevated.
- A free bone flap is created using a high-speed drill.
- The dura is opened in a circular fashion based on tumour, location and size.
- The aim of excision of a convexity meningioma is to achieve complete macroscopic resection of the tumour, including the dural and bony attachments. This may necessitate taking a margin of dura of approximately 1 cm surrounding the tumour. Tumour resection is based on the Simpson grading system (Figure 3.6).
- The tumour is devascularized by isolating the blood supply and performing an internal debulk. This may be achieved by using the CUSA.
- Once you have identified the arachnoid plane, the tumour is then dissected off the surrounding brain.
- The tumour is then imploded and removed in a piecemeal fashion.
- Careful attention is paid to the arachnoid plane at the tumour–brain interface to ensure no residual tumour is left behind. Resection of the involved dura and bone may be required.
- Ensure adequate haemostasis.

Convexity meningioma

Key points and safety considerations
Location of craniotomy – Image guidance

Resection of the dural tail.

Discussion of Simpson grading.

Identification of arachnoid plane and preservation of arteries.

Potential pitfalls

Drilling of a hyperostotic (meningioma infiltration) calvaria.

Defining the exact anatomical location.

Case 19

A 68-year-old woman presents with headaches, progressive unilateral visual loss and anosmia. Her MRI scan demonstrated a diffuse densely enhancing tumour arising from the anterior skull base with the anterior cerebral arteries located posterior to the lesion and the optic chiasm located inferior to the lesion. She has been scheduled for surgery.

Olfactory groove meningioma

- Pre-operative steroids and antibiotics are given, and a urinary catheter is inserted.
- The patient is placed supine with the head fixed on a Mayfield three-point pin headrest.
- The head is neutral with 20° neck extension for subfrontal approach; the head is rotated 30° contralaterally for pterional approach.
- Bicoronal or pterional scalp incision is used, depending on the approach.
- A square of pericranium is preserved and reflected.
- Large tumours (>3 cm) are approached by a bifrontal craniotomy, then subfrontal approach. The sagittal sinus and falx are divided anteriorly. Small tumours are approached by unilateral subfrontal or pterional approach; if midline, the right side is preferred.
- For a unilateral approach, three burr holes are made.
  - One in the midline.
  - Two laterally at the root of zygomatic process of the frontal bone.
- Care is taken not to enter the bony orbit.
- Using a high-speed drill, a free bone flap is fashioned.
- If the frontal sinus is opened, the mucoperiosteum is stripped away and packed with Betadine-soaked gauze. (This will be removed at the end of the operation.)
- A 3–4 cm linear incision of the dura is made over each medial inferior frontal lobe.
- The bridging veins are coagulated and divided.
- Frontal lobe is carefully retracted laterally and posteriorly to expose the tumour.
- The tumour is devascularized by isolating the blood supply (e.g. ethmoidal arteries) at the base of the tumour.
- The tumour is internally debulked by using the CUSA.
- Once the arachnoid plane is identified, it is then dissected off the surrounding brain tissue.
- Preserve the anterior cerebral artery (ACA) branches, which may be encased by the tumour.
- The tumour is then imploded and removed piecemeal.
- Careful attention is paid to the arachnoid plane at the tumour–brain interface to make sure that no residual tumour is left behind (including involved dura and bone).
- If the frontal sinus has been breached, the posterior wall should be drilled away and periosteum laid over.
- Ensure adequate haemostasis.

Olfactory groove meningioma

Key points and safety considerations

Anatomical description of olfactory groove, planum sphenoidale and tuberculum sellae.

Location and control of anterior (and posterior) ethmoidal arteries.

Limitations of techniques to preserve olfaction.

Protection of possible adherent ACA branches.

Decompression of optic canals if extension distally around optic nerves.

CSF repair (addressing the frontal sinus, pericranial flap and 'pros and cons' of lumbar drains).

Potential pitfalls

Attaining early control of blood supply depends largely on your chosen approach (e.g. transbasal approach).

If describing techniques such as extended endoscopic endonasal or supracilliary minicraniotomy techniques, make sure that the given lesion is suitable for such an approach and be prepared to demonstrate awareness of their difficulties and limitations.

Case 20

Considerations in selecting operative approaches for tuberculum sellae/planum sphenoidale meningiomas

The discussion would involve the extended trans-tubercular endoscopic endonasal transsphenoidal (EEETS) approach vs. the transcranial approaches. The potential advantages of the EEETS are the following: avoidance of excessive manipulations on the neural structures including the chiasma, early drilling of skull base bone and dural origin achieving a more radical resection and early devascularization of the tumour, in larger lesions on the planum control of the posterior ethmoidal artery result in further devascularization (beware this artery is near Cranial Nerve II and avoid heat injury during coagulation), early visualization of the superior hypophyseal artery offering avoidance and better preservation of visual function. In the exam settings, it is an important demonstration of safety as a priority. Be aware of the limitations and complication avoidance with the EEETS approach. The limitations (depending upon an experience which is not expected from a candidate sitting the exam) include large lesions with encasement of major vessels, extension lateral to the ICA, lateral extension beyond the mid-pupillary line or extension retroclival into interpeduncular cistern. Specific complications include increased risk of CSF leak and anosmia (may be minimized by exceptional techniques). Therefore, it is important to adequately study the pre-operative images looking for the size and extent of the lesion, 'cortical cuff' between the edge of tumour and major vessels, calcification and consistency as judged by the T2-weighted signal on MRI. Perhaps in many cases, the extension of the meningioma into the optic canal would favour transcranial approaches. Although this can be determined pre-operatively by the imaging or the pattern of visual deficits, in the majority, these are apparent on opening and exploration of the optic canal. Through an EEETS approach, drilling and opening of the optic canal is feasible and access medial to the optic nerve; however, extension into the supero-medial segment of the optic canal would be less accessible.

For a pterional craniotomy approach, the area medial to the ipsilateral optic nerve is a blind spot necessitating some manipulation of that nerve and if it is already compromised may result in ipsilateral visual deterioration. Furthermore, the branches of the superior of hypophyseal artery would be obscured. It remains debateable to add an extradural anterior clinoidectomy, a step with potential morbidity, in every case prior to opening the dura. An anterior interhemispheric approach in selected cases would allow resection of the tumour and opening of both optic canals (in most cases, incision of the falciform ligament is sufficient to access the optic canal as the proximal bony roof is deficient) without manipulations of the optic nerves or chiasma. Also, early visualization of the superior hypophyseal artery is an advantage.

Case 21

A 58-year-old woman presents with a chronic history of headaches and now reports an unsteady gait. Her MRI scan demonstrated a frontotemporal dural-based tumour with the lesion abutting the Sylvian fissure with a local mass effect. She has been scheduled for surgery.

Sphenoid wing meningioma

- Pre-operative angiogram with embolization may be required.
- Pre-operative steroids and antibiotics are given and a urinary catheter is inserted.
- The patient is placed supine with the head rotated to 30–45° to the opposite side and secured in a Mayfield three-point pin headrest.
- Mild extension (15–30°) aids in temporal lobe retraction.
- Fronto-temporal curvilinear skin incision is made extending 1 cm anterior to the tragus to 1 cm behind the hairline.
- A myocutaneous flap is reflected in one layer.
- A burr hole is placed in the keyhole region. Ensure the orbit is not entered.
- Another burr hole is placed just above the zygoma.
- A free bone flap is fashioned.
- A Budde halo is then assembled.
- Using a high-speed drill, the hyperostosis of the greater wing of the sphenoid is drilled until flush with the middle cranial fossa floor.
- The dura is opened in a curvilinear fashion (leaving a cuff wide enough to wall off epidural bleeding and aid in dural closure), reflected and tacked with sutures.
- The tumour is devascularized by isolating the blood supply and performing an internal debulk by using the CUSA.
- Once the arachnoid plane is identified, the tumour is then dissected away from the surrounding brain tissue.
- Pay particular attention to the opercular segment of the MCA, anterior clinoid artery, carotid artery, optic nerve and the cavernous sinus. In particular, clinoidal meningiomas extend to suprasellar region and tends to encase optic nerve, ICA, A1 and M1 with the lenticulostriate braches being most liable to injury in these cases.
- The area is covered with cottonoids.

- The tumour is then imploded and removed piecemeal.
- Careful attention is paid to the arachnoid plane at the tumour–brain interface to make sure that no residual tumour is left behind (including dura and bone).
- Ensure adequate haemostasis.

Case 22

A 56-year-old woman presents with headaches, dizziness and new onset of seizures. Her MRI scan demonstrates a parafalcine dural-based lesion in the parietal lobe. She has been scheduled for surgery.

Parafalcine meningioma

- Pre-operative angiogram with embolization may be required.
- Pre-operative steroids and antibiotics are given, and a urinary catheter is inserted.
- The patient is placed supine with the head fixed on a Mayfield three-point pin headrest.
- The head is then elevated to approximately 30°.
- When using the image guidance system, the tumour may be identified and marked on the patient's scalp.
- A large reversed U-shaped flap is used. (Incorporate an additional 1 cm margin from the tumour edge.)
- Several burr holes are made over the superior sagittal sinus (SSS). Using a craniotome, a free bone flap is created.
- The SSS is separated under direct vision.
- The exposed SSS is covered with cottonoids and Surgicel.
- Tack-up sutures are placed before opening the dura.
- The dura is opened circumferentially around the tumour with the dural base on the SSS.
- The tumour is devascularized by isolating the blood supply and internally debulked by using the CUSA.
- Identify the arachnoid plane. The tumour is then dissected away from the surrounding brain. The area is covered with cottonoids.
- The tumour is then imploded and removed piecemeal.
- Careful attention must be paid to the arachnoid plane at the tumour–brain interface to make sure that no residual tumour is left behind (including dura and bone).
- Ensure adequate haemostasis.

Parasagittal/parafalcine meningioma

Key points and safety considerations

Image guidance.

Placement of craniotomy over the midline – safe burr holes (perforator over sinus vs. paramedian burr holes and drilling over the sinus).

Preservation of the draining veins.

Protection of anterior cerebral arteries deep to the tumour.

Total vs. near-total resection, if the sinus is invaded.

Potential pitfalls

Depending on imaging to establish sinus patency.

In cases of sinus occlusion, wide falcine resection compromises collateral venous channels within dural leaves.

Resection of infiltrated sinus and reconstruction. (Even in most expert hands, significant precautions should be observed. This operation may not be considered an option in the posterior half.)

Case 23

A 36-year-old woman presents with a chronic history of headaches. Her MRI scan demonstrates uniform enhancement of a space-occupying lesion in the lateral ventricle with mild hydrocephalus. She has been scheduled for surgery.

Intraventricular meningioma (posterior parieto–occipital transcortical approach)

- Pre-operative angiogram with embolization may be considered.
- Pre-operative steroids and antibiotics are given, and a urinary catheter is inserted.
- The patient is placed in a park bench position with the head secured in a Mayfield three-point pin fixation and elevated approximately 30°. When using the image guidance system, the tumour may be identified and marked on the patient's scalp.
- In selecting an entry point, the superior parietal eminence is often optimal.
- A reverse U-shaped incision is used.
- A free bone flap is created.
- A Budde halo and microscope are used.
- The trajectory into the ipsilateral ventricle may be identified using an image guidance system and confirmed using a Dandy drainage cannula. Describe the anatomy of overlying white matter tracts and in particular the optic radiation.
- Internal decompression of the tumour is performed using microsurgical techniques.
- A CUSA may help to minimize brain retraction.
- Occlusion of the choroidal artery branches should be achieved as early as possible.
- Careful attention is paid to the arachnoid plane at the tumour–brain interface to make sure that no residual tumour is left behind.
- Ensure adequate haemostasis.
- An EVD is inserted and remains *in situ* for the next 24 hours.

Case 24

A 48-year-old woman presents with thoracic pain and progressive lower limb weakness. She now walks with a stick. Her spinal MRI scan demonstrated an intradural extramedullary spinal tumour. She has been scheduled for surgery.

Debulking of an intradural spinal lesion (meningioma)

- Pre-operative level marking may be performed by a radiologist.
- Pre-operative steroids and antibiotics are given, and a urinary catheter is inserted.

- Intraoperative neurophysiology monitoring is recommended.
- The procedure is performed in a prone position on a Wilson frame, Montreal mattress or Jackson table. Pressure points are well protected.
- A linear midline incision is performed over the marked area.
- Both paraspinous muscles are stripped with monopolar diathermy.
- A laminectomy is performed, ensuring the cranial and caudal end of the tumour is exposed. The tumour is usually visible underneath the arachnoid.
- The operating microscope is brought into the operative field.
- If the tumour is not visible, ultrasonography may be beneficial to evaluate the margins of the tumour. If inadequate exposure is seen, additional bone is removed to provide unobstructed surgical access.
- A linear durotomy is made and dural edges are hitched.
- The extent of the tumour is again examined.
- The tumour capsule is then coagulated with low-voltage bipolar diathermy.
- The arachnoid is sharply divided and reflected to allow internal decompression of the tumour using either bipolar suction or CUSA.
- The plane between the tumour and spinal cord is then developed with progressive infolding of the tumour edges.
- Circumferential dissection in the arachnoid plane is continued until the tumour capsule is delivered in its entirety.
- The dural base is coagulated or excised.
- Adequate haemostasis must be ensured.

Resection of spinal meningioma

Key points and safety considerations

Correct localization of anatomical level.

Avoidance of manipulations of the spinal cord.

Possible benefits of intraoperative neurophysiological monitoring for extramedullary lesions.

Potential pitfalls

Consider division of the adjacent denticulate ligaments or sacrifice of a dorsal thoracic nerve root to gain access to an anterolaterally placed lesion rather than manipulating or retracting the spinal cord.

Prepare to discuss the case 'for or against' resection of the dural origin (e.g. true risk of recurrence vs dural repair and CSF leak).

Principles of operative surgery and surgical anatomy

In-Depth Topics

Here, we discuss some topics where more nuanced discussions may be required, which go beyond the simple step-by-step details of an operation.

A. Principles of intracranial aneurysm clipping

The emhasis is on safety and complication avoidance.

Position

Take into account the inclination of the skull base. Elevate the head. Avoid kinking of the jugular veins. Assess the degree of rotation and the location of the aneurysm to allow the temporal lobe to 'fall' away by gravity. For example, the position is more vertical for a laterally projecting posterior communicating artery (PCoA) aneurysm in order not to approach the fundus first and the position is more horizontal for a posteriorly projecting PCoA aneurysm in order to visualize the medial aspect of the aneurysm neck.

Craniotomy

Craniotomy should be large enough to allow access, angulations and different trajectories for the aneurysm clip. Usually, a more frontal exposure is required. Drill the sphenoid wing to minimize brain retraction. If you select a superciliary minicraniotomy (not recommended in an exam setting), then be prepared to address a premature aneurysm rupture and describe the use of special aneurysm clip applicators.

Brain relaxation

Lumbar drain

Beware of contraindication in the presence of associated intracranial haemorrhage (ICH).

EVD insertion

The EVD can be opened once the dura is opened to drain CSF from the basal cisterns. Drainage of CSF after incision and opening of the basal cisterns is the most common and effective way to achieve brain relaxation.

Ventricular puncture

Direct intraoperative ventricular puncture by aspiration of CSF should be considered, especially in the presence of ventriculomegaly and a swollen brain precluding access to the basal cisterns. The frontal horn is deep at the level of the inferior frontal gyrus. During a pterional craniotomy, the puncture point is 1–2 cm superior and 2–3 cm anterior to the anterior Sylvian point.

ICH evacuation

In the presence of a parenchymal ICH, partial evacuation of the haematoma, without eliminating the tamponade effect on the ruptured aneurysm, helps to achieve brain relaxation to access the basal cisterns and to achieve proximal control.

Basal cisterns

Opening the basal cisterns to drain CSF is important to help achieve brain relaxation.

Avoid brain retraction

Retraction injury should be avoided by adequate brain relaxation and CSF egress. Retractors, if used, act as brain 'holders' with only minimum pressure applied. Sharp dissection should be performed (e.g., splitting the Sylvian fissure). The direction of retraction and mobilization should be cautious in the following situations: (1) temporal lateral retraction in cases of laterally pointing PCoA aneurysms and (2) frontal superior retraction in cases of large inferiorly pointing ACoA aneurysms. In the former, the fundus may be adherent to the medial temporal lobe, and in the latter, the aneurysm may be adherent to the optic chiasm and lead to premature rupture.

Proximal control

This step must be mentioned in describing the overall procedure. In cases of MCA aneurysms, splitting of the Sylvian fissure widely exposes the M1 segment for proximal control. This also provides access to other territories (trans-Sylvian approach) and minimizes brain retraction. Special care should be given to preserving the perforators. In cases of temporary clip application, the perforators should be carefully dissected adjacent to the parent vessel to avoid their inclusion into the clip blades. For example, apply the temporary clip to the M1 distal to the origin of the lenticulostriate artery and in cases of applying the temporary clip to the A1 artery avoid inclusion of the recurrent artery of Heubner.

Neck dissection, clip application and preservation of distal branches

The identification of the aneurysm neck allows for clip placement and reduction in perforator injury. The aneurysm clip should be applied following full dissection of the aneurysm neck after adequate space is made for the insertion of the clip blades. An attempt to use the clip blades to dissect aneurysm may result in rupture or tearing of the aneurysm sac. The manufacturers indicate that the closing pressure is less at the tip of the blades. Ensure that the clip blades are beyond the aneurysm neck. Multiple clip reconstruction may be required for wide-necked aneurysms. In selected cases, the use of appropriate fenestrated clips avoids kinking of distal branches and potential slippage. The clip should occlude the aneurysm, and allow patency of perforators and major branches. Intraoperative indocyanine green (ICG) fluorescence angiography is valuable in assessing aneurysm exclusion and vessel patency.

Temporary clip application

During an intraoperative rupture, the application of temporary clips is necessary. They can also be used during the steps of neck dissection, particularly with friable aneurysms that are adherent to surrounding vessels. The temporary clip decreases the tension and slackens the sac to facilitate successful clip application. The closing pressure of temporary clips is less than for the definitive clip. Nevertheless, avoid application of the clip on a parent vessel with an atheromatous segment because this may lead to a plaque 'break' and formation of thromboembolism. Preserve the perforators. When clipping an M1 aneurysm, avoid compromising the lumen of the MCA branches, including the lenticulostriate arteries. Likewise, when clipping an A1 aneurysm, preserve the recurrent artery of Heubner. In cases of prolonged temporary clip application, ensure neuroprotection: head elevation, maintenance of perfusion blood pressure and adequate oxygenation and sedation (e.g., mannitol and propofol). In cases of SAH, the tolerability is variable and depends on the vulnerability of neural tissue and the vessel itself (less tolerated for the basilar artery aneurysm). The duration of temporary clip application may be guided by monitoring techniques, such as SSEPs.

Avoid intraoperative aneurysm rupture

Measures to avoid rupture include anaesthetic techniques, limited brain retraction, proximal control, application of temporary clips and proper dissection of the aneurysm neck. Ensure that the patient remains haemodynamically stable. Maintain a stable blood pressure with appropriate anaesthesia and adequate analgesia. The anatomy of the aneurysm should be appreciated. For example, aggressive temporal retraction may result in premature rupture of a laterally projecting PCoA aneurysm with its fundus adherent to the temporal lobe. In addition, superior retraction on the frontal lobe may tear an inferiorly projecting ACoA aneurysm with fundus adherent to the optic chiasm or optic nerve. Complete the neck dissection prior to clip application. Perform sharp dissection of arachnoid adhesions to prevent the clip blades from tearing the fundus. Apply a temporary clip if the aneurysm sac appears tense. Intraoperative rupture can occur during any stage of the operation. This is most challenging if it occurs before access to the parent vessel. This will necessitate aggressive anaesthetic measures to combat brain swelling in order to obtain control. Moreover, neuroprotection is also required with prolonged temporary clip application. Full identification and dissection of the aneurysm neck is required – a hasty clip application may lead to premature rupture.

B. Principles of intrinsic glioma resection

The emphasis is on understanding the neuro anatomy, recent technical advances and controversies.

Image-guidance systems

Image-guidance systems are used routinely in neurosurgery. To establish a histological diagnosis, image-guided biopsies are performed. Image guidance helps the surgeon to select the shortest route from the cortical surface, avoid traversing the ventricular cavities and vascular areas (e.g., Sylvian fissure and pineal region) and eloquent areas. In cases of glioma resection, image guidance helps to confirm the underlying anatomy, delineate tumour margins and demonstrate white matter tracts (with the use of tractography).

Awake craniotomy

Different anaesthetic techniques including local anaesthesia and sedation or 'asleep – awake – asleep' techniques using general anaesthesia with intraoperative wake-up can be used. Electrophysiological mapping includes frequency of stimulation, cortical and white matter tract stimulation, and speech and motor assessments. Awake craniotomy is safe and well tolerated. Be aware of the safety topics: airway protection, avoidance and management of intraoperative seizures (cold saline), vomiting and pain control. Be prepared to debate the merits of this approach compared to other options (intraoperative MRI).

Intraoperative monitoring

Resection of intrinsic lesions is a favourite exam question, which assesses your neuroanatomical knowledge. Describe the lesion in relation to the sulcus and gyrus. The choice of trajectory is selected to indicate your anatomical knowledge, including eloquent areas and white matter tracts. Intraoperative monitoring is a surgical adjunct to aid in your resection. Demonstrate knowledge of the neurophysiological parameters, frequency of stimulation, design of the bipolar stimulators and types of recordings. For example, motor responses are recorded by clinical assessment or neurophysiological monitoring. Speech responses (including higher mental function) require experienced neurologists, neuropsychologists or speech and language therapists. You should be aware of the variation in amplitude and frequency of stimulation in assessing the white matter tracts. You should express your knowledge of the anatomy, orientation and projection of the white matter tracts.

Ultrasound

Ultrasound uses high-frequency sound waves to create an image. The advantages include availability and real-time imaging. Disadvantages include surgeon dependence and limited resolution.

5-Aminolevulinic acid

5-ALA is a porphyrin-based compound that does not cross an intact blood–brain barrier and is selectively taken up into malignant glial cells. The 'dye' is activated with light at the near-blue spectrum and fluoresces by emitting wavelengths near the red spectrum. It is detected by filters mounted on the operative microscope.

Cavitron ultrasonic surgical aspirator (CUSA)

The ultrasonic waves induce shock waves, bubbling and cavitation to the intracellular water content coupled with expansion, evaporation and disruption of cells. CUSA can be selected for firm lesions to help reduce intraoperative bleeding and perioperative morbidity. CUSA has a limited value in debulking extremely calcified or dense fibrous lesions. The heat generated may also be detrimental to the adjacent neural structures.

Gliadel wafers

There has been a recent change in practice. Although less commonly used, you may be asked to describe their chemical composition (polifeprosan 20 with carmustine implant), relative contraindications (open ventricles), potential side effects (e.g., seizures, brain oedema, delayed wound healing and intracranial infections) and indications in newly diagnosed and recurrent high-grade malignant gliomas. Be aware of the surgical techniques of placement of the wafers and the importance of dural closure.

C. Considerations in the surgical management of craniopharyngiomas

The discussion regarding these cases in the exam setting is centred around your decision-making process based on evidence base and safe practice. Do not just embark on radical resection. You should be aware of the controversies for this topic and the variable considerations. These are a few points to help guide your preparation to tackle this topic:

- The different patterns (mostly in radiological studies) include cystic components, calcification, extensions into different compartments and ventricles, location in relations to the stalk (e.g., pre- or retro-infundibular) and encasement of neurovascular structures. Other factors to be considered include pattern of visual dysfunction, endocrine function, neurological status and age. They determine surgical procedures such as minimal approaches including stereotactic cyst drainage with possible insertion of an Ommaya reservoir or insertion of intracystic catheters for drug administration such as interferon, subtotal resections with or without upfront radiotherapy or the feasibility of more radical resection. There are specific considerations to determine the choice of the surgical approach; the most important is to avoid breaching the integrity of an intact third ventricular floor; otherwise, hypothalamic dysfunction with all its sequelae arise, avoid damaging the visual pathways especially the blood supply by the branches of the superior hypophyseal artery and avoid blind dissection of the component extending into the interpeduncular cistern with possible injury to the basilar artery perforators. The surgical procedures range from extended endonasal endoscopic approach to pterional, anterior interhemispheric, subfrontal and transcallosal approaches. Multicompartmental extension, calcification, encasement of neurovascular structures, purely intraventricular location, extension to interpeduncular cistern, visual deficit pattern indicating either superior chiasmal or optic tract compression would favour a transcranial over an endoscopic endonasal approach.
- The important safety issue to discuss is addressing hydrocephalus and methods of CSF diversion including endoscopic septostomy for single-shunt insertion. These may be combined with an endoscopic procedure such as biopsy or decompression of a cystic component within the ventricle.
- There are differences in managing craniopharyngiomas in the paediatric and adult age groups. These determine the extent and timing of resection, use adjuvant radiotherapy, the surgical approach, the implications of long-term sequelae and follow-up. Examples of these include different pathological entities (adamantinomatous vs. papillary) with different molecular biology types and potential therapeutic targets. The effect of resulting hypopituitarism on the growing patient may determine deferment of radical procedures until growth is completed. The non-aerated SS (until age of 5 years) may preclude endonasal endoscopic approaches (it is possible to overcome this challenge with image guidance). The long-term complications such as the risk of diabetes may dictate extending the follow up to adulthood. Similarly, the late effects of radiation (if used) need to be considered.
- The realistic figures in relation to avoidance of post-treatment DI even with anatomical preservation of the stalk. The difference between the DI resulting

from stalk division vs. hypothalamic injury may include adipsic DI, which is problematic to manage.

- Recurrent cases are less likely to be radically excised by repeat surgery and are associated with higher operative morbidity. Therefore, justification of less radical safer approaches and complementary adjuvant treatment is reasonable.

D. Principles of microsurgical resection of arteriovenous malformations

Operative planning

Review the imaging (MRI scan and angiogram) to assess the nidal anatomy, obtain critical information regarding the major feeding vessels and draining veins, identify arteries *en passage* and establish if a cortical AVM is based on the ventricle.

Compartments

Arterial

The angiogram assesses the filling of the nidus by different vascular territories demonstrated by different injections. Do not rely on one injection. On reviewing the carotid injection, it is possible to underestimate the extent of the AVM if it is supplied by distal MCA or ACA branches.

Venous

Multiple draining veins are common. However, in a few cases, compartmentalization of the nidus may occur with each segment predominantly draining into a different draining vein. Pre-operatively, the appreciation of this arrangement allows for the surgeon to plan to expose all the draining veins and allow for complete resection.

Nidus location

The location of the nidus determines the 'eloquence' of the AVM and predicts the patient's potential post-operative neurological deficits. An MRI scan demonstrates its relationship to the cortical regions and plans the trajectory (e.g., transsulcal approach for subcortical lesions). The AVM's relationship to white matter tracts can be seen by tractography, and its relationship to functional neural tissue can be seen by fMRI imaging. One limitation of fMRI imaging is that the signal adjacent to the abnormal blood flow through the nidus may be difficult to determine.

Feeders

Knowledge of angiographic anatomy enables the surgeon to determine the location of the main feeders (e.g., the two terminal branches of the PCA are located in the calcarine and occipito-parietal sulci).

Draining veins

Knowing the location of the surface draining veins is the key to intraoperative localization of the nidus. The location of the deep venous drainage would identify the deep extent of the nidus.

Craniotomy

Plan the craniotomy. A large flap is recommended in the following instances:

- AVM nidus cannot be retracted as much as the surgeon would often like.
- The nidus cannot be gutted from within.
- The surface veins may further restrict one's access to the base of the malformation.
- Adequate identification of surface clues are needed.
- The draining vein on the surface needs to be traced retrogradely to locate the subcortical nidus.

Skeletonization of vessels

The initial dissection aims to access the arterial feeders, identify the draining veins and access the nidus. The covering arachnoidal membrane has to be meticulously incised to expose the adequate segments of the vessels circumferentially.

Identification of draining veins

The arterialized draining veins are initially preserved because premature occlusion of these veins may result in significant and troublesome bleeding secondary to an increase in the intranidal pressure. The veins act as a 'gauge'. Their collapse and colour change (returning to venous dark blue) indicate adequate obliteration of the nidus, and only then can the AVM be disconnected and subsequently removed.

Resection of nidus

Cautery and interruption of feeding vessels are required. Use bipolar coagulation perpendicular to the vessels. Ensure that you are constantly moving around the AVM to ensure that your dissection is performed evenly (avoid deep holes). Apply Surgicel and cottonoids to help establish the brain–AVM interface. Once the dissected cavity is a few centimetres deep, place a temporary clip on the major feeder to help establish that it is terminating in one nidus. This will also help decrease the tension within the AVM. In addition, cortical AVMs are based on the ventricle. Secure the ventricle and address the choroidal and ependymal feeders. Once the test occlusion is complete, a permanent aneurysmal clip is placed on the main draining vein.

En-passage feeders

These feeders should be respected, perhaps leaving a temporary clip and only dividing the feeders that terminate in the nidus.

Finale

Ensure adequate haemostasis throughout the surgery. Small feeders that are not adequately coagulated may retract and result in parenchymal intracerebral haematoma. Test the resection bed for breakthrough bleeding. Breakthrough bleeding can be evidence of retained AVM or disrupted autoregulation in the surrounding tissue. Persistent bleeding from the AVM bed usually indicates a residual nidus. In such cases, the nidus should be explored and resected accordingly.

E. Principles of trauma craniotomy

Craniotomy

For small and moderate acute subdural and extradural haematomas, the craniotomy should be tailored to encompass the margins of the haematoma. In cases of fracture haematomas, the craniotomy should circumscribe areas of a comminuted skull fracture to allow the bone fragments to be fixed together with mini-plates.

For large subdural and extradural haematomas associated with diffuse head injuries, a large frontotemporoparietal craniotomy allows for adequate decompression of the haematoma, haemostasis and brain swelling.

Acute extradural haematoma

This surgical procedure is expected to be described in detailed during the examination. Be aware of the challenging questions related to the techniques for bleeding (including intraoperative coagulopathy), brain swelling, dural laceration and torn sinuses.

Acute subdural haematoma

Acute subdural haematomas are commonly associated with severe head injuries. The traumatic forces disrupt the underlying brain tissue and the bridging veins. The haematoma can be associated with underlying brain contusions (including a 'burst' temporal lobe). In these cases, a decompressive craniectomy is required to address the haematoma, brain swelling and increased intracranial pressure.

Contusions

Contusions can be located deep and superficial to the brain's surface. Deep-seated contusions that extend to the cortical surface may incorporate viable and functional neural tissue. Cortical location and time from injury have implications in surgical planning. In cases of multiple contusions and persistent increased intracranial pressure, a decompressive craniectomy may be considered.

Intraoperative swelling

Intraoperative swelling can occur throughout surgery: at the time of dural opening, clot evacuation or closure. In these cases, recommend the following:

- Elevate the patient's head.
- Optimize the anaesthetic parameters (ensure adequate oxygenation, ventilation and sedation; treat with mannitol and brief moderate hyperventilation).
- Effect rapid evacuation of the haematoma.
- Coagulate bleeding vessels.
- Assess for a reversible cause – residual haematoma. If ultrasound is available, this may identify a deep intracerebral ICH or, rarely, an interhemispheric subdural haematoma.
- Leave the dura open (with or without a dural substitute).
- Check to see if insertion of an ICP bolt and immediate post-operative CT scan is recommended.

F. Principles of specialized disorders

Movement disorders

- Ensure knowledge of the disorder: The clinical features, pathophysiology, neurotransmitters and management.
- Know the principles of stereotaxy and the different types of stereotactic frames.
- Plan target and trajectory: Stimulation in awake patients, stereotaxic atlases, Tesla (3T) MRI imaging including tractography and microelectrode recordings.
- Know the surgical steps: Create burr hole, open dura and pia maters, advance electrode (check impedance), ± obtain electrode recordings and stimulation and implant deep brain stimulation (DBS).

Epilepsy

- Operative planning includes the following:
  - Confirmation of the diagnosis (e.g., exclude pseudoseizures).
  - Establishing indications for surgery (frequency, quality of life, medical intractable seizures).
  - Localize the focus (non-invasive vs. invasive grid and depth electrodes).
  - List types of surgery (palliative, resections and stimulation).
  - Review investigations: Imaging (MRI, fMRI, PET, ictal and interictal SPECT), Wada testing, neuropsychological testing and electroencephalographic (EEG) findings.
- Demonstrate knowledge regarding neuroanatomical principles of temporal lobectomy, extratemporal resections, subpial transections, vagal nerve stimulator (VNS) insertion, anatomy and approaches to choroid plexus, choroid fissure, hippocampus and amygdala. Discuss surgery outcome scales.

Engel epilepsy surgery outcome scale

- *Class I*: Free of disabling seizures.
- *Class II*: Rare disabling seizures ('almost seizure-free').
- *Class III*: Worthwhile improvement.
- *Class IV*: No worthwhile improvement.

Spasticity

- Demonstrate knowledge regarding aetiology, pathophysiology, grading systems (see Table 3.3) and treatments of spasticity.
- Medical options include diazepam, baclofen, dantrolene and progabide.
- Surgical options include botulinum injections, intrathecal baclofen, electrical stimulation via epidural electrodes, selective dorsal rhizotomy, intramuscular phenol neurolyis, myelotomies, stereotactic thalamotomy or dentatomy.

G. Carotid artery stenosis

- Demonstrate awareness of evidence-based trials regarding the indications for carotid endarterectomy: Asymptomatic Carotid Surgery Trial (ACST), Asymptomatic Carotid Atherosclerosis Study (ACAS), Veterans Affairs

Table 3.3 Ashworth grading system for spasticity

Grade	Description
0	No increase in muscle tone.
1	Slight increase in muscle tone, manifested by a catch and release or by minimal resistance at the end of the range of motion when the affected part(s) is moved in flexion or extension.
1+	Slight increase in muscle tone, manifested by a catch, followed by minimal resistance throughout the remainder (less than half) of the range of movement (ROM).
2	More marked increase in muscle tone through most of the ROM, but affected part(s) easily moved.
3	Considerable increase in muscle tone, passive movement difficult.
4	Affected part(s) rigid in flexion or extension.

Cooperative Study (VACS), European Carotid Surgery Trial (ECST) and North American Symptomatic Carotid Endarterectomy Trial (NACET) (for full details, see Chapter 7: Landmark Publications).
- State anatomical landmarks and important structures encountered during the procedure, including platysma, fascial planes, carotid sheath, carotid arteries (common, external and internal), carotid sinus, recurrent laryngeal nerve, vagus nerve, marginal mandibular branch of facial nerve, ansa cervicalis and hypoglossal nerve.
- Discuss intraoperative monitoring: Transcranial Doppler (TCD) and EEG.
- Note controversies: Selective or routine intraoperative intraluminal shunting, patient selection and carotid artery stenting.

H. CSF leakage
- State aetiology of CSF leakage including cranial and spinal pathology (traumatic, spontaneous, congenital, iatrogenic, medication [dopamine agonists]).
- Discuss pre-operative imaging: CT and MRI.
- List principles of CSF surgical repair.
  - Cranial approaches: Craniotomy and endoscopic intranasal approach and the use of intraoperative dyes (fluorescein) during the repair.
  - Spinal approaches: Open repair and shunting (e.g. lumbar drain).
- Do not forget to use prophylactic Pneumovax, when appropriate.

I. Peripheral neuropathies
- Definitions
  Peripheral neuropathy: Diffuse lesions of peripheral nerves producing weakness, sensory disturbance and/or reflex changes.
  Mononeuropathy: A disorder of a single nerve, often attributed to trauma or entrapment.
  Mononeuropathy multiplex: Involvement of two or more nerves, usually due to a systemic abnormality.
- Aetiology of peripheral neuropathies. Use the mnemonic: **ABCDEFGHI**

A	Alcoholism, Amyloid, AIDS, Acute intermittent porphyria
B	B12 deficiency
C	Chronic inflammatory demyelinating polyneuropathy, Connective tissue disorders (polyarteritis nodosa, rheumatoid arthritis, systematic lupus erythematosus)
D	Diabetes, Drugs (vincristine, dexamethasone, statins, metronidazole, phenytoin, amitriptyline), Diphtheria
E	Endocrine, Entrapment, Environmental toxins (organophosphate)
F	Thyroid disorders (hypothyroidism – carpal tunnel syndrome, hyperthyroidism – polyneuropathy)
G	Guillain–Barré syndrome
H	Hereditary (Charot-Marie-Tooth disease)
I	Infection (Leprosy – Hansen's disease)

- The clinical features of the following neuropathies are important: Brachial plexus injuries, median nerve entrapment, ulnar nerve entrapment and radial nerve entrapment (Figure 3.7).
- Classification of peripheral nerve injuries: Seddon system (1943) and Sunderland system (1951) (see Table 3.4).

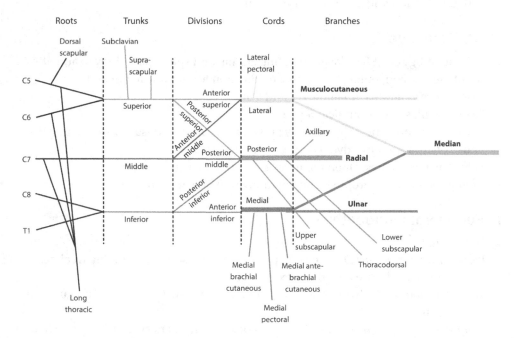

Figure 3.7 Schematic diagram of the brachial plexus.

Table 3.4 Peripheral nerve injuries: Seddon and Sunderland classifications of peripheral nerve injury

Sunderland	Seddon	Description of injury	Recovery period
I	Neurapraxia	Conduction block, nerve is in-continuity, Wallerian degeneration does not take place	≤ 3 months
II	Axonotmesis	Axon not continuous, nerve itself remains intact, axonal sprouting, Wallerian degeneration	1 inch [25.4 mm] per month
III		During healing, excessive scarring of the endoneurium occurs that hinders axon regeneration	< 1 inch per month where it is slowed by the scar tissue; determined by degree of scarring and involved fascicles
IV		Nerve is still in-continuity, scar build-up blocks nerve regeneration	Surgical intervention is required to re-establish nerve transduction by removing scar tissue and reconnecting nerve segments
V	Neurotmesis	Rupture of the nerve, it is no longer a continuous fibre	Recovery requires surgical intervention

- *Nerve growth factor* (*NGF*) is a secreted protein that promotes differentiation, growth, maintenance and survival of certain target neurons. They have an important role in signalling, neuroprotection and repair.

Summary and Advice

- **The emphasis of this section of the examination is your neuroanatomical knowledge, safety and complication avoidance.**
- **Straightforward cases should require straightforward answers. For example: Carpal tunnel decompression, lumbar microdiscectomy or craniotomy for an extradural heamatoma.**
- **For many candidates, this section of the exam may allow them to gain maximum points.**

4 | The Viva: Investigation of the Neurosurgical Patient

Introduction

This section of the exam should cover familiar territory. Being quizzed on investigations is a daily occurrence during neurosurgical training. Therefore, there is an expectation that your exam performance will be smooth and structured. A large proportion of this section will be radiology but bear in mind other investigations (e.g. nerve conduction studies, neuropathology, audiometry and perimetry).

In a Viva setting, please remember this is a neurosurgical rather than a radiology examination. Imagine that you are communicating the results of radiological investigations with a neurosurgeon over the telephone in order to determine a patient's treatment options. Describe the radiological images to establish the differential diagnosis, the anatomical location of the lesion (deep vs. superficial), ease of surgery, possible complications and timing of surgery based on mass effect and herniation.

When describing an image, it is important to state the type of investigation and verify the patient's demographic details and date of this investigation. For computed tomography (CT) and magnetic resonance imaging (MRI) scans, report the imaging modality and plane (e.g. axial, coronal or sagittal) and describe whether the lesion is intra- or extra-axial. Describe if the scan is with or without contrast. If contrast is given, is there evidence of contrast enhancement? This will narrow the list of differential diagnoses. Be precise about the anatomical location of the lesion. It is best to avoid general terms, such as 'brainstem'; be specific: for example, 'the lesion is in the left side of the tegmentum of the midbrain at the level of the inferior colliculi.' Similarly, in the cerebrum, locate the lesion by its lobe, gyrus, sulcus and most importantly its neurological function. Proximity to motor cortex or Broca's area should also be emphasized. In addition, for deep-seated lesions, mention the adjacent white matter tracts. This will allow your management to be safe and clear (surgical vs. non-surgical management; biopsy vs. subtotal vs. total resections; and potential complications of treatment). Include descriptions of mass effect, perilesional oedema and hydrocephalus.

DOI: 10.1201/9781003254379-4

MRI scan interpretation – Sample answer

This axial MRI scan T1-weighted image without contrast demonstrates a large solitary well-defined heterogeneous/variable intensity mass in the right/left frontal lobe adjacent to ____. There is also associated surrounding oedema and mass effect as evidenced by the sulcal effacement and compression of the ____ ventricle. These features are suggestive of ____, although other differentials include____. (See Table 4.1 for the differential diagnosis of intracranial lesions.)

Targeted differential diagnosis

Having studied tables and lists of differential diagnoses from neurosurgical textbooks, you may be surprised that when shown a radiological image the vast majority of the list of differential diagnoses do not apply. Starting your answer with 'There are many possibilities to explain this image…' and then finding out that there are only two potential diagnoses may lead to a difficult situation. For example, the list of differential diagnoses of a vascular blush on a cerebral angiogram includes vascular malformations, dural arteriovenous fistula (DAVF), renal cell metastases, haemangiopericytoma or haemangioblastoma. However, if the angiogram depicts a large arteriovenous malformation (AVM) in the parietal lobe, with feeding arteries leading to a tangled nidus that shunts blood directly into a large draining vein, there is only one diagnosis. Therefore, it is best to provide a short list of possible differential diagnoses and explain your reasoning.

Management justification

This is not a separate exam component, but rather it is one of the purposes, if not the main purpose, of oral and clinical examination. Management is an important feature in the investigation Viva. Therefore, after formulating a diagnosis, treatment options should be discussed. It is best to list all the treatment modalities (e.g. conservative, medical, radiological and surgical) and then place emphasis on the most important treatments. In the Viva, presenting a balanced view may be a challenge. Do not appear hesitant or flippant. Remember, it is best to recommend safe and standard treatment options.

Principles of radiology

In this section, you may also be asked about the principles of radiology.

- CT scan.
- MRI scan.
- Single-photon emission computed tomography (SPECT) scan.
- Positron emission tomography (PET) scan.

- **CT scan** – It utilizes an X-ray beam, which traverses the patient's head, and a diametrically opposed detector that measures the extent of resorption. Use the terms hypodense, isodense and hyperdense.
- **MRI scan** – A strong magnet causes protons in the body to align with that field. When a radiofrequency current is applied the protons spin out of equilibrium. When the radiofrequency filed is turned off the time the protons take to realign and the energy they give off depends on their physical properties which can be translated into an image. Use the terms hypointense (low signal), isointense and hyper-intense (high signal).

Table 4.1 Differential diagnosis of intracranial lesions based on anatomical location, +/− enhancement and +/− surrounding oedema

Location		Enhancement	Lesion	Oedema
Supra-tentorial	Extra-axial	+	Meningioma	±
		+	Metastasis	+
		−	Arachnoid cyst	−
		−	Epidermoid cyst	−
	Intra-axial	+	High-grade glioma	+
		+	Pilocytic astrocytoma	
		+	Metastasis	++
		+	Cerebral lymphoma	+
		−	Low-grade glioma	−
	Sella/suprasellar	+	Pituitary adenoma	−
		+	Craniopharyngioma	±
		−	Rathke's cleft cyst	−
		±	Optic nerve glioma	±
	Intra-ventricular	+	Colloid cyst	
		+	Glioma/central neurocytoma	N/A
		+	Meningioma	N/A
		+	Choroid plexus papilloma	N/A
		+	Ependymoma	N/A
		+	Subependymoma	N/A
Infra-tentorial	Extra-axial	+	Meningioma	±
		+	Schwannoma	
		−	Epidermoid cyst	−
	Intra-axial	+	Metastasis	++
		+	Medulloblastoma	+
		+	Pilocytic astrocytoma	−
		+	Haemangioblastoma	−
		+	Brainstem glioma	±
	Intra-ventricular	+	Ependymoma	N/A
		+	Choroid plexus papilloma	N/A

- T1 – **Spin-lattice relaxation**. The time taken for protons to realign themselves with a magnetic field.
- T2 – **Spin-to-spin relaxation**. The time taken for protons to return to their out-of-phase state.
- **Diffusion weighted** – Thermally driven translational movement of water. The same principle can be used to produce **diffusion tensor imaging** (**DTI**) to outline white matter tracts.
- **Functional** – T2 relaxation time of perfused brain – oxyHb. A mismatch of O_2 supply and utilization in the activated area causes signal change due to blood-oxygenation-level-dependent (BOLD).
- **Perfusion** – Bolus tracking after rapid contrast injection.
- **SPECT scan**
  - Uses compounds labelled with gamma-emitting tracers.
- **PET scan**
  - Utilizes positron-emitting isotope bound compound.
  - Need a cyclotron for production.
  - To assess the relationship of cerebral blood flow (CBF) and O_2 demand.
- **Ultrasound**
  - Uses high-frequency sound waves to image soft tissue to produce a real-time moving image. Use the term hyper- or hypo-echoic. The technique may be used in children prior to their sutures fusing. Coronal or sagittal images may be seen. It is not possible to have axial images.

Notes on particular MRI sequences

- Remember **T1-weighted images** are 'anatomical', e.g. grey matter is grey and white matter white. In **T2-weighted images**, this is reversed. The only things that appear bright on T1 are fat, melanin, gadolineum and subacute blood. Some say that T2 is more for 'pathology'. This, of course, is particularly true in the spine where the hyper-intense CSF highlights very clearly compression of the hypointense neural structures.
- One should always say whether the scan is with **contrast** or not. Look for enhancement of nasal mucosa and the dural venous sinuses if contrast is given.
- **Fluid attenuated inversion recovery** (**FLAIR**) images are still T2 weighted, but the CSF signal has been suppressed so it appears black. The scans shown in Figures 4.1 and 4.2 are similar, as CSF is black in both, but the image on the left shows an 'anatomical' arrangement with the grey matter being grey and white matter being white. This arrangement is reversed on the image on the right and is therefore a T2-weighted scan, but given that CSF is black, it must be FLAIR.

Another pair of sequences that must be understood contains **diffusion-weighted imaging** (**DWI**) and **apparent diffusion coefficient** (**ADC**) map. DWI is characterized by only a faint outline of the scalp and skull. The brain stands out much more clearly. CSF can be either white or black, depending on the b value. ADC maps are characterized by a very pixelated appearance with the scalp being visible. The two sequences must be looked at in combination. A lesion may be said to be restricting diffusion (of water molecules) if there is a **high signal on DWI** with a corresponding **low signal on ADC**. Lesions that restrict include cerebral infarction, abscess, active

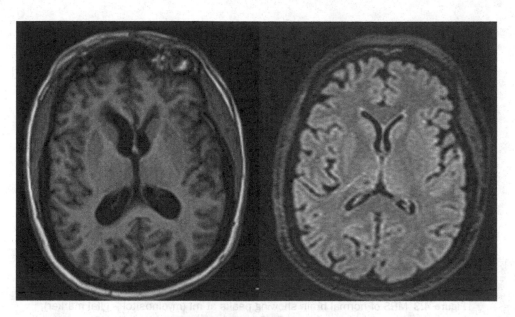

Figure 4.1 T1WI (left), FLAIR (right).

MS plaque and some tumours (e.g. lymphoma, ependymoma, some meningiomas). This list is by no means exhaustive. In the exams, there are several scenarios that come up repeatedly: tumour vs. abscess in the cerebrum, epidermoid vs. arachnoid cyst in posterior fossa and low-grade glioma vs. infarction.

- **Three-dimensional constructive interference in steady state (CISS) studies** reduce CSF pulsation artefact and provide excellent visualization of cranial nerve anatomy and small membranes such as the floor of the third ventricle. CISS is the term used by Seimens. It has other names according to manufacturers including FIESTA (GE). It is a strongly T2-weighted gradient echo sequence.

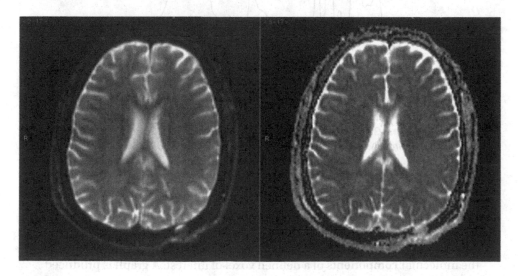

Figure 4.2 DWI (left), ADC (right).

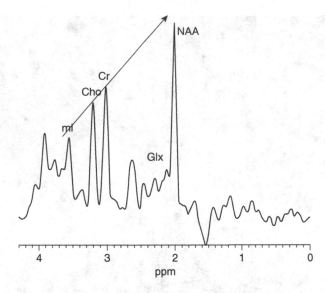

Figure 4.3 MRS of normal brain showing peaks at ml (myoinositol – glial marker), Cho (Choline – membrane marker), Cr (Creatine – energy marker), Glx (Glutamate – neurotransmitter) and NAA (N-acetyl aspartate – neuronal marker). The angle formed is called Hunter's angle. In a high-grade glioma, the angle is reversed (see Figure 4.4) due to an elevated Cho due to increased membrane turnover and reduced NAA due to loss of neurones.

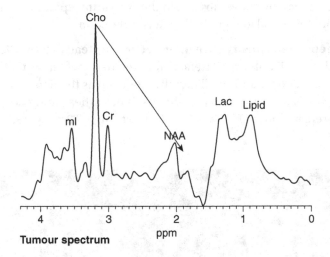

Tumour spectrum

Figure 4.4 Tumour spectrum. (Adapted from Guidelines for Acquiring and Reporting Clinical Neurospectroscopy, November 2012, *Seminars in Neurology* 32(5): 557–558. DOI: 10.1055/s-0033-1336414.)

- **Susceptibility-weighted imaging (SWI)** is also known as T2* or gradient echo. It is a form of T2WI which is susceptible to **iron or calcium**. Most useful in highlighting haemorrhage, e.g., subtle subarachnoid haemorrhage (SAH) or haemorrhagic lesions such as cavernomas. These areas stand out as being very dark.
- **Magnetic resonance spectroscopy (MRS)** uses particular software to analyse the molecular components of a defined voxel of interest. A graph is produced showing characteristic peaks (Figures 4.3 and 4.4).

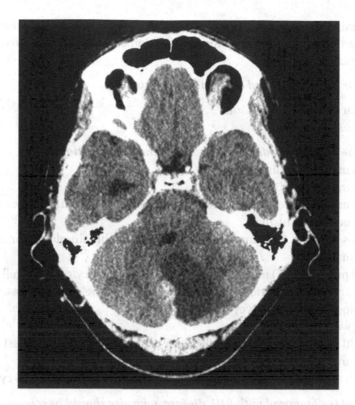

Figure 4.5 CT Head scan (Case 1).

Case scenarios

Case 1

A 35-year-old woman presents with acute worsening headaches with a background history of progressive lower limb weakness. Her Glasgow Coma Scale (GCS) was 15/15 (Figure 4.5).

Please describe the anomaly shown.
This axial CT scan demonstrates a left cerebellar cystic lesion with an enhancing mural nodule and compression of the fourth ventricle. There is evidence of surrounding oedema. The right temporal horn appears rather enlarged.

Tips

You may also mention this:

'I would also like to review the rest of the axial images to assess for hydrocephalus'.

Remember, this patient has headaches and progressive lower limb weakness. Why? The next question could be the following.

What could have been the cause for her presentation?
- Headache: Hydrocephalus, posterior fossa mass, other supratentorial haemangioblastoma.

- Paraparesis: It is difficult to explain these symptoms from the cerebellar lesion alone; perhaps a concurrent motor cortex lesion or spinal cord lesions should also be included.

What is your provisional and differential diagnosis?

- Cerebellar haemangioblastoma.
- Pilocytic astrocytoma.

What are the relevant clinical examinations and investigations?

- Assessment of cerebellar signs.
- Assessment of lower limb weakness.
- Time permitting, assess for possible von Hippel–Lindau (VHL) with enquiry into the patient's family history.
  - Fundoscopy and slit-lamp examination by the ophthalmologist for retinal angiomas.
  - Blood pressure (BP) measurement for phaeochromocytoma, as well as 24-hours urine collection for catecholamines and their metabolites.
  - Full blood count for polycythaemia.
- Imaging would include:
  - An MRI scan of the whole neuroaxis for concurrent haemangioblastoma in the brain and spinal cord and endolymphatic sac tumour?
  - A CT scan of thorax/abdomen/pelvis for solid organ tumours and cyst.

If the patient is diagnosed with VHL disease, who else should be screened?

- All first-degree relatives should be screened. The guidelines are based on the age of the patient (Figure 4.6).
  - An undiagnosed adult will be screened for all of these conditions.
  - It is important to arrange genetic counselling and educate the patient on VHL.
- If she plans to become pregnant, involve an obstetrician and highlight the relevance of contraception, pre-implantation genetic counselling and termination (if appropriate).

On her spinal MRI scan, multiple avidly enhancing lesions were seen. How would you manage these lesions?

Guide the management on clinical and radiological features. If the lesions were causing progressive paraparesis, then the discussion should be focused on resection of the relevant lesions; otherwise, surveillance at regular intervals depending on the clinical picture is recommended.

If this haemangioblastoma was found incidentally, how would you approach the situation?

Discuss the options with the patient and family and screen her for VHL. It is essential to be guided by a complete neurological examination whilst looking for early signs of cerebellar and brainstem compression. Given an option, surgical resection is preferred because there is evidence of fourth ventricular compression and possible hydrocephalus.

Case 2

A 36-year-old woman, who is 24-weeks pregnant, presents with persistent headaches, vomiting and bilateral papilloedema. She is alert and orientated (Figure 4.7).

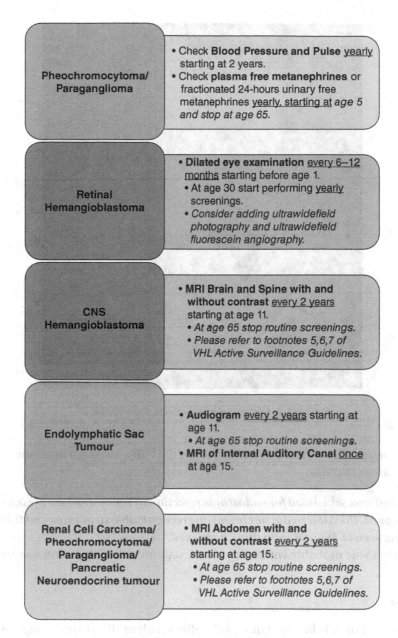

Pheochromocytoma/ Paraganglioma
- Check **Blood Pressure and Pulse** <u>yearly</u> starting at 2 years.
- Check **plasma free metanephrines** or fractionated 24-hours urinary free metanephrines <u>yearly, starting at</u> *age 5 and stop at age 65.*

Retinal Hemangioblastoma
- **Dilated eye examination** <u>every 6–12 months</u> starting before age 1.
- At age 30 start performing <u>yearly</u> screenings.
- *Consider adding ultrawidefield photography and ultrawidefield fluorescein angiography.*

CNS Hemangioblastoma
- **MRI Brain and Spine with and without contrast** <u>every 2 years</u> starting at age 11.
- *At age 65 stop routine screenings.*
- *Please refer to footnotes 5,6,7 of VHL Active Surveillance Guidelines.*

Endolymphatic Sac Tumour
- **Audiogram** <u>every 2 years</u> starting at age 11.
- *At age 65 stop routine screenings.*
- **MRI of Internal Auditory Canal** <u>once</u> at age 15.

Renal Cell Carcinoma/ Pheochromocytoma/ Paraganglioma/ Pancreatic Neuroendocrine tumour
- **MRI Abdomen with and without contrast** <u>every 2 years</u> starting at age 15.
- *At age 65 stop routine screenings.*
- *Please refer to footnotes 5,6,7 of VHL Active Surveillance Guidelines.*

Figure 4.6 Guidelines for VHL monitoring.

What is the diagnosis?
This is an axial MRI of the head that shows a hyper-intense lesion at the level of the foramen of Monro, causing biventricular hydrocephalus. This is most likely due to a colloid cyst.

What would your management options be?
The key clinical problems are the following:

1. The patient is facing a life-threatening condition secondary to hydrocephalus.
2. She is pregnant with a viable fetus. There is a need for an urgent multi-disciplinary discussion with the obstetrician (foetal-maternal specialist), neonatologist, obstetric anaesthetist and intensivist. If the patient's condition

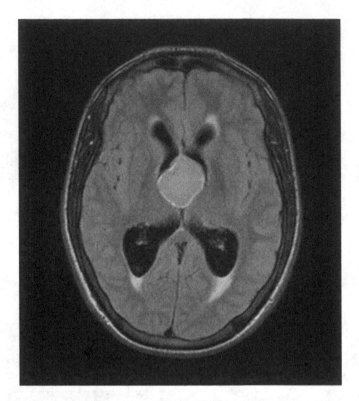

Figure 4.7 MRI Head scan – axial slice (Case 2).

deteriorates, there is an option of delivering the baby, although prematurely, with a caesarean section.

The patient was scheduled for endoscopic resection of the cyst. When the introducer was removed, the camera did not reveal any recognizable structures and there were no visible vessels. What do you think happened?
The camera was probably within the cavum septum pellucidum and needed to be readjusted.

Case 3

A 25-year-old man is involved in a road traffic accident (RTA) and brought into the emergency department comatose (Figure 4.8).

Please identify the intracranial pressure (ICP) waveforms.
The third wave from the top.

What is the abnormality here? Please describe what each peak may represent.
The P2 is greater than P1: This would represent a non-compliant brain in a high ICP setting (intracranial hypertension).

- P1: Percussion wave represents arterial pulsation.
- P2: Tidal wave represents intracranial compliance.
- P3: Dicrotic wave represents aortic valve closure.

In healthy patients, the height of P1 > P2 > P3.

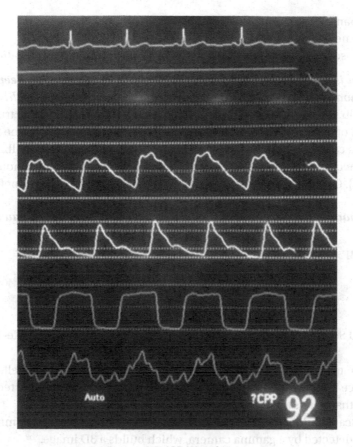

Figure 4.8 ICP Waveforms.

What are the possible methods of ICP measurements?

Clinical monitoring is very important and reliable.

- The most common method in a neurosurgical setting is with an ICP monitor. This can be achieved by direct methods of measurement using an intraventricular device, e.g., using an external ventricular drain (EVD) and attaching it to a transducer (the gold standard, which has therapeutic advantages).
- Other methods include the use of microtransducer devices and placing them in the following areas:
  - Parenchyma (most common).
  - Subarachnoid.
  - Subdural.
  - Epidural and lumbar spine.
- The devices used are broadly divided into the following:
  - Piezoelectric strain gauge devices (Codman).
  - Fibreoptic (Camino).
  - Pneumatic sensors (Spiegelberg).

The pneumatic device does not need zeroing and calibrates itself every hour. There is a potential risk of zero drifting that may affect the accuracy of the device.

- Indirect methods of measurement can be used as well.
  - Transcranial Doppler (TCD).

- Tympanic membrane displacement.
- Optic neural sheath diameter.
- Fundoscopy (Frisen scale), although this requires prolonged elevation of ICPs.

The patient is in the intensive care unit (ICU) and ventilated with deep sedation. What method of cerebral oxygenation determination could be used in this situation?
Jugular bulb oximetry uses fibre-optic technology to detect the spectrum of light absorption of oxyhaemoglobin. Alternatively, a jugular puncture can be performed or a venous catheter could be passed to place the tip on the jugular bulb. This could be performed on the side of brain injury where there is dominant venous drainage (debatable). Cerebral oximetry (near-infrared spectroscopy) can be beneficial.

What methods of measurement of cerebral blood flow (CBF) are you aware of?

$$CBF = \frac{\text{cerebral perfusion pressure (CPP)}}{\text{cerebrovascular resistance (CVR)}}.$$

- Clinical examination and consciousness level (GCS).
- TCD.
- Kety and Schmidt's method is based on the Fick principle using an Xe-133 CT scan.
- PET scan to measure a specific body process or function. A radiolabelled substance is injected into the body. Positrons are released and detected by a camera that builds a three-dimensional (3D) image.
- SPECT scan: Radioactive substance that measures CBF – releases gamma rays that are detected by a gamma camera, which builds a 3D image.
- CT perfusion.
- MR perfusion.

What other direct method of measurement could be used to measure cerebral metabolism in this patient?
Microdialysis utilizes Ringer's lactate at the rate of 0.3 µL/minutes through a semi-permeable membrane. The dialysate is extracted and assessed for the following products: lactate, glycerol, glucose and glutamate. A lactate/pyruvate ration >25 is an early warning of ischaemia and mitochondrial dysfunction.

Case 4

A 50-year-old woman with known renal failure presents with a sudden severe headache (Figure 4.9).

Please describe this non-contrast scan. What is the diagnosis and the differential diagnosis?
This plain CT head scan demonstrates a large heterogeneous right-sided globular-shaped mass with evidence of peripheral calcification. There is some fresh haemorrhage that has extended into the ventricular system. The mass effect and bleed appear to have occluded the right foramen of Monro, causing contralateral dilated ventricles. There is an abnormal projection from the mass posteriorly; a giant

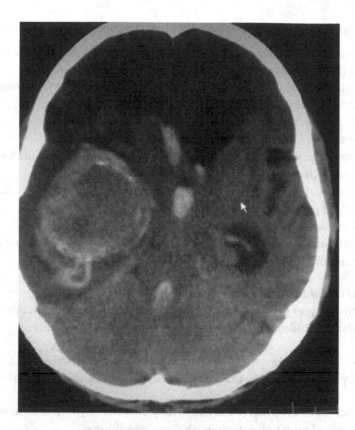

Figure 4.9 CT Head scan (Case 4).

aneurysm should be considered as a primary diagnosis. The differential diagnosis would also include haemorrhagic tumour (primary or secondary).

What other types of imaging may help to diagnose the condition?
CT angiogram/digital subtraction angiogram.

The lesion was treated surgically with a high-flow bypass and clipping. How would the patient be followed up as an outpatient?
She can be followed up with serial scans. The available options are computed tomography angiogram (CTA), magnetic resonance angiography (MRA) +/− digital subtraction angiography (DSA). This selection would depend on the local hospital's policy because all are acceptable methods with their own merits and risks. Because the patient had surgical treatment, based on the ISAT trial, there is a lower incidence of recurrence as compared to coiling. It may be preferable to perform MRA using the time of flight (TOF) sequence, which eliminates the risk of contrast nephropathy because this patient has renal failure.

The patient became more drowsy on day 5 after surgery. What are the relevant investigations necessary in this situation?
Obtain a complete history, assess the vital signs and perform the clinical examination. Further bedside assessments include arterial blood gases (ABGs), BP, temperature and fluid balance.

The following causes, with their appropriate investigations, should be considered:

- Hyponatraemia secondary to syndrome of inappropriate antidiuretic hormone secretion (SIADH) or cerebral salt wasting (CSW) – Serum sodium.
- Pneumonia or pulmonary emboli secondary to inadequate oxygenation and lung complications – ABG and electrocardiography (ECG).
- Urinary tract infection (UTI) – Urine microscopy.
- Hydrocephalus – Urgent CT brain scan.
- Re-haemorrhage secondary to hyperperfusion breakthrough or failed vascular anastomosis – Urgent CT brain.
- Delayed cerebral ischaemia and infarction from inadequate bypass – SPECT scan, CT/MRI perfusion and MRI with DWI.
- Cerebral vasospasm – TCD.
- Seizure (non-convulsive/convulsive) – Electroencephalography (EEG) and SPECT scan for interictal images.

How is TCD useful in aneurysmal rupture?
TCD uses the Doppler principle and can measure the following: heart rate (HR), peak volume, pulsatility index, end-diastolic velocity and Lindegaard ratio.

Lindegaard ratio = mean velocity in the middle cerebral artery (MCA) divided by mean velocity in ipsilateral extracranial internal carotid artery (ICA)

- High velocities in the MCA (>120 cm/s) may be due to hyperaemia or vasospasm.
- The Lindegaard ratio helps distinguish these conditions:
  - <3: Hyperaemia.
  - >3: Vasospasm (3–6: mild; >6: severe).

Three main windows are used: the temporal, suboccipital and orbital.

In approximately 10% of patients, a temporal window produces inadequate insonation (ultrasound cannot penetrate the temporal bone).

The artery is identified by the direction of flow and depth.

- MCA: 6 cm and flow towards the probe at 55 cm/s.
- ACA: 5 cm flow away from the probe at 50 cm/s.
- PCA: 5 cm and flow towards the probe with a velocity of 40 cm/s.

The patient's identical twin sister is concerned about having a similar lesion herself and is keen to be investigated. How would you advise her?
In general, one reserves screening for patients with two or more first-degree relatives who had subarchnoid haemorrhages. However, it is not unreasonable to consider a scan. There is a slight increase in aneurysm incidence among identical twins. However, there are merits and disadvantages. A screening tool, such as a CTA, may be done. The scan is not 100% sensitive in identifying all aneurysms, and therefore, a small proportion could be missed that could potentially rupture in the future. Because the natural history of aneurysm is still poorly understood, a negative scan does not mean that an aneurysm will not develop in the future. An aneurysm that is found may not rupture. However, a positive finding may put the clinician and patient in a dilemma because treatment itself is not risk free. The level of anxiety may increase, and this may affect the patient's lifestyle, occupation, driving, travel, insurance and

so forth. With a positive result, the patient may undergo serial imaging, which carries a risk of radiation. There is no clear consensus on how an aneurysm may be managed, although there are guidelines. The treatment options are surgery or endovascular embolization. Some patients may be simply monitored.

The risk of bleeding from unruptured aneurysms is provided by the ISUIA study, PHASES score and a multi disciplinary consensus on the unruptured aneurysm treatment score.

Case 5

A 46-year-old teacher was admitted to the neurosurgical ward with a recent onset of cognitive decline and headache. An MRI brain scan demonstrates a contrast-enhancing solitary lesion adjacent to the occipital horn of the left ventricle. She underwent a frameless-based biopsy of the underlying lesion.

Describe the histology slide.
This slide demonstrates an area of hyper-cellularity with marked hyperchromatism and pleomorphism. There is also prominent vascularity and an area of palisading necrosis.

What is the diagnosis?
Glioblastoma multiforme (Figure 4.10).

Explain the WHO Classification of Tumours of the Central Nervous System (2021)?
The fifth edition of the WHO Classification of Tumours of the Central Nervous System (CNS), published in 2021, is the sixth version of the international standard for the classification of brain and spinal cord tumours. This new classification introduces major changes that advance the role of molecular diagnostics in CNS tumour classification. At the same time, it remains loyal to other established approaches to tumour diagnosis such as histology and immunohistochemistry. New tumour types and subtypes are introduced; some are based on novel diagnostic technologies such as DNA methylome profiling.

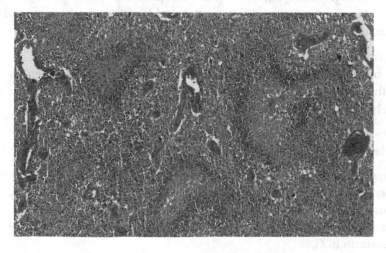

Figure 4.10 Histology (Case 5).

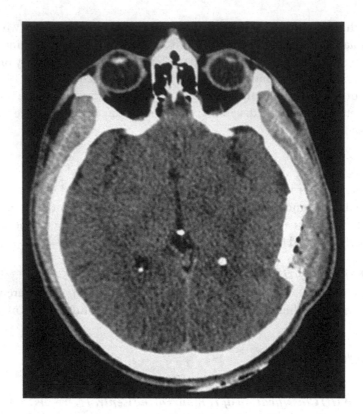

Figure 4.11 CT Head scan (Case 6).

Case 6

A 26-year-old newsreader was assaulted and presented with a GCS of 13/15 (E3V4M6) (Figures 4.11 and 4.12).

Where is the abnormality? What is the immediate management?
The patient has a depressed skull fracture in the left temporo-parietal region. There is a small contusion underlying the fracture. This patient requires a complete primary and secondary survey. Based on the anatomical location, the fracture and haematoma consider starting the patient on anticonvulsants.

There was no wound. How would you manage this patient?
I would be guided by the patient's neurological status. Because there is no open wound, this is not a neurosurgical emergency. This may be potentially managed conservatively. I would engage the patient in this decision.

What neurological deficits could be present?
Right-sided hemiparesis and dysphasia.

The patient was managed in the ICU and was localizing to pain; however, he had regular episodes of unexplained neurological deterioration. How would you investigate this?
Consider nonconvulsive seizures; check the patient's serum glucose, serum sodium and perform an EEG.

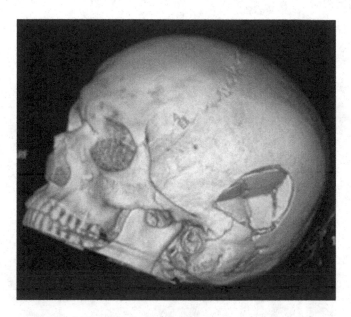

Figure 4.12 CT Head scan – Reconstruction (Case 6).

There was a new onset of progressive dysphasia. A repeat CT scan demonstrated localized oedema. His family was inquiring if surgery could be helpful in reversing this and controlling seizures.

Surgery (e.g., elevating a depressed skull fracture) could be undertaken for progressive neurological deficit, and this may reverse. However, there is no convincing evidence about improving seizure control.

He was discharged home and presented 6 weeks later with an episode of generalized seizure. What are the possible causes for this event?

The patient may be developing late-onset post-traumatic seizures (PTS) secondary to his head injury. Other possibilities are intracranial abscess, subdural empyema and venous sinus thrombosis.

Case 7

A 13-year-old girl presents with worsening gait and frequent falls at school (Figure 4.13).

What is the abnormality?

A split cord abnormality with a median septum (type 1 diastematomyelia).

What is the diagnosis?

Split cord malformation (SCM).

Why could the patient be experiencing neurological deterioration?

During growth spurts, patients may deteriorate as a result of pressure on the spinal cord.

What pre-operative investigations and imaging are necessary?

- Complete MRI imaging of neuraxis.
- CT myelography.

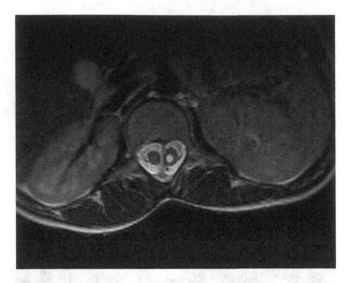

Figure 4.13 Spinal MRI scan (Case 7).

- An MRI of abdomen at the level of the lesion (SCM may be associated with neurenteric cyst).
- Urodynamic testing.

The patient was found to have a low-lying conus medullaris. Why is this important from a surgical point of view?

There may be an associated tethered cord. This is important because the spinal team may be considering scoliosis correction, and it would require neurosurgical involvement.

There are two different situations that need to be addressed: a tethered cord and the diastometomyelia.

Which should be treated first and why?

It is safer to treat the SCM first. If detethering the cord is performed instead, there is a risk of the cord shearing when it moves cranially through a rigid bony septum.

If this were an isolated incidental finding, would it need treatment?

This is controversial. Because some centres do not operate unless there is a neurological deficit or progressive neurological deficits. Some may offer surgery before any symptoms develop. Both approaches have advantages and disadvantages. Some would prefer to operate at the earliest sign of neurological deficit. The patient would need to be seen regularly in the clinic and her parents would need to be counselled on this management.

Case 8

A 40-year-old man presents 3 weeks after a motor vehicle accident with a facial injury and unilateral red eye (Figure 4.14).

What are the possibilities?

- Carotid-cavernous fistula (CCF) with chemosis and ophthalmoplegia. Examine for bruit, pulsatile exophthalmos and increased intraocular pressure.

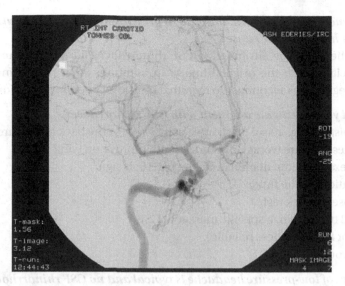

Figure 4.14 Cerebral Angiogram (Case 8).

- Ocular injury and infection.
- Sinusitis and ophthalmitis.

Describe the findings seen in the image.

This digital subtraction angiogram (DSA) carotid injection image demonstrates dilatation of the superior ophthalmic vein and coil embolization.

How do you classify this condition?

Barrow classification for CCF is as follows.

A. Direct high-flow shunt between the ICA and cavernous sinus. Often develops from ruptured cavernous ICA aneurysm.
B. Indirect low-flow dural shunts between meningeal branches of the ICA and the cavernous sinus.
C. Indirect low-flow dural shunts between meningeal branches of the external carotid artery (ECA) and the cavernous sinus.
D. Indirect low-flow dural shunts between meningeal branches of both the ICA and ECA and the cavernous sinus.

What are the factors that would influence your management of this patient?

- High flow.
- Increased intraocular pressure.
- Symptomatic visual deterioration.
- Progressive proptosis.
- On DSA, cortical venous filling.
- Intractable bruit.

What could be performed?

Attempt a coil embolization. The coils could be placed on the feeding artery and/or in the draining superior ophthalmic vein itself.

Following successful treatment, the patient presents later with postural headaches. What could have been the cause?

His headaches could be attributed to CSF rhinorrhoea causing low-pressure headaches associated with the original injury. In addition, other causes include autonomic dysregulations secondary to hypothalamic injury and hypotension.

How would you investigate a patient with CSF rhinorrhoea?

- Obtain history: e.g., nasal discharge ('salty water in the back of the throat') and headaches (that are worse on standing and improve on lying down).
- Clinical examination: demonstrate the reservoir sign.
- Investigations of the fluid:
  - Glucose dipstick test.
  - Beta-2 transferrin, a specific marker of CSF.
  - Ring or halo sign (less reliable).
  - Tau protein.

If the history of low-pressure headache is typical and no CSF rhinorrhoea is identified, what would your management be?

Investigate for leaking CSF along the neuroaxis with a fine-cut CT scan/CT myelography. Involve the ENT surgeons to consider nasoendoscopy with fluorescein dye.

Reference

Barrow DL, Spector RH, Braun IF, et al. Classification and treatment of spontaneous carotidcavernous fistulas. *J Neurosurg* 1985; 62: 248–256.

Case 9

A baby is brought to the emergency department by her mother after a fall that occurred 3 days ago. There was a large swelling over the vertex (Figure 4.15).

Could you identify the normal and abnormal structures? Describe the fracture, sutures and vascular markings.

The fracture is more radiolucent than the other sutures, has no serration along its edges and is blind ending. At the blind end, it is more tapered than at the sutural or proximal end. Vascular markings are less straight and have branches.

Upon stabilization and admission, please state the key steps involved in the patient's management. What are other investigations that may be necessary?

- Neurological monitoring.
- Activation of the hospital's child protection team. Non-accidental injury (NAI) must be assumed in all such cases.
- CT scan to exclude a chronic subdural haematoma (may not be performed if the child is stable).
- Ophthalmic review for retinal haemorrhage.
- Skeletal survey for old healed fractures.

How would you clinically assess her for increasing ICP?

- Consciousness level (GCS).
- Anterior fontanelle pressure.

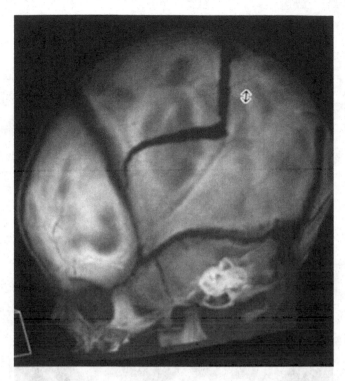

Figure 4.15 Radiological imaging (Case 9).

- Head circumference.
- Measuring the height at which the fontanelle begins to sink (crude estimate).

Her CT head scan demonstrates a small haematoma deep to the fracture. How would you manage this?
At this stage, the patient would be managed conservatively because the GCS remains stable. There is a significant risk of haemorrhage from surgery, particularly bleeding from the superior sagittal sinus.

The mother is a Jehovah's Witness, and does not agree to blood product transfusion for her child during surgery. How would you take this forward?
If the child requires surgery, discuss the options and involve the child protection team, senior colleagues and hospital solicitors and discuss the options again with the mother. If all fails, this matter could be referred to the court.

The patient was discharged and 6 months later presents with progressively enlarged swelling over the vertex. What could this be?
Leptomeningeal cyst (growing fracture).

Case 10

A 45-year-old woman was brought to the emergency department in a state of stupor after 4 days of neck pain (Figure 4.16).

What is the most likely diagnosis?
Left-sided cerebellar infarction with obliteration of the fourth ventricle. Consider cerebellar metastasis with surrounding oedema.

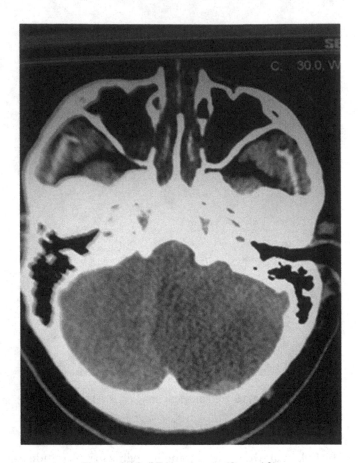

Figure 4.16 CT Head scan (Case 10).

What other images would you like to see?
An MRI scan with contrast and DWI (including the supratentorial compartment to assess for hydrocephalus) and a CTA scan.

What would be your immediate management?
Have a brief discussion with the family for history and assess the overall condition of the patient. In the meantime, prepare the patient for surgery. If the patient has gross hydrocephalus, insert an EVD followed by wide suboccipital craniectomy and foramen magnum decompression is recommended.

The patient recovers well following surgery with a GCS of 14 (E4V4M6). She was noted to have left-sided partial ptosis and unequal pupils. What could have been the cause?
This could be secondary to disruption of the sympathetic flow secondary to Wallenberg syndrome. (Be prepared to list the other components.) Establish from the patient's history if this was congenital or pre-existing.

The neurologist is keen to start the patient on anticoagulants as soon as possible. When would you consider this safe?
Provided there is no contraindication such as expanding haematoma (ruled out with up-to-date CT scan), anticoagulation may be commenced. However, it is important

to balance the benefits and potential risks (including bleeding). A further discussion with the family is recommended.

Case 11

A 46-year-old farmer presents with progressive spastic paraparesis (Figures 4.17 and 4.18).

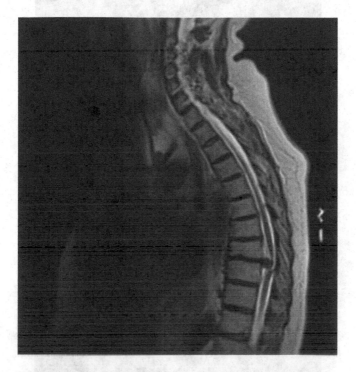

Figure 4.17 Spinal MRI scan – sagittal slice (Case 11).

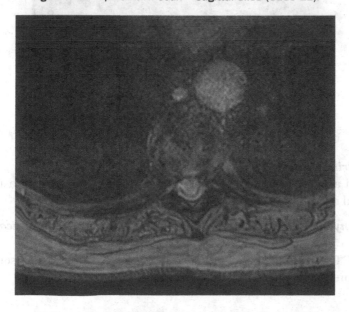

Figure 4.18 Spinal MRI scan – axial slice (Case 11).

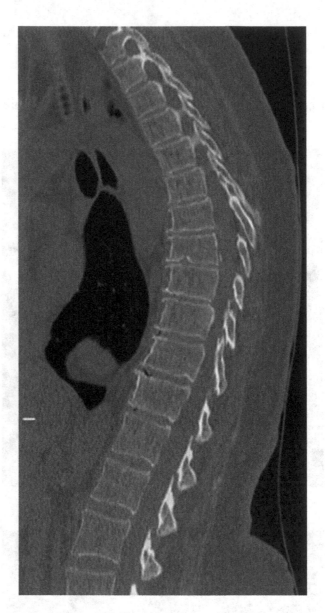

Figure 4.19 Thoracic CT scan (Case 11).

Please describe the MRI scan.
Sagittal and axial T2-weighted MRIs of the midthoracic region demonstrate a very large central disc prolapse with severe cord compression.

Are there any other imaging modalities to assist you with your surgical planning and why?
A thoracic CT scan should be requested to look for calcification. If present, it makes the operation significantly more difficult (Figure 4.19).

Please describe the CT scans below.

CT scan showing sagittal views of the thoracic spine. There is only a small fleck of calcification at the level of the disc prolapse.

What are the surgical options?

There should be recognition that this is a difficult case requiring an inter-disciplinary input. One should be clear that posterior decompression would not be a good idea, even in a patient who is declining quickly. Approaches are based on the laterality of the disc. In this case, being central, approaches such as costotransversectomy, transpedicular and transfacetal would be challenging. A transthoracic approach would be indicated. One might consider the option of endoscopic, if expertise is available. Use of intraoperative monitoring may also be useful.

For a transthoracic approach, what are the key parts of the operation?

- *Anaesthesia*: Placement of double-lumen tube.
- *Positioning*: Lateral with the table broken.
- *Localization*: Possibly the most vital part of the operation. Preoperative placement of a radio-opaque marker is extremely useful (e.g., tantalum beads in the pedicle, etc.), otherwise 'counting from below' – again vital that there is a pre-operative thoracolumbar MRI. A cervicothoracic MRI scan is not good enough. The patient's shoulder will prevent counting from above, and there are irregularities in the number of thoracic vertebrae.
- *Approach*: Often together with cardiothoracic colleagues. Portion of rib head may need to be resected. Drilling of rib head and anterior end plates above and below disc space. Delivery of disc into space created. There may be mention of the artery of Adamkiewicz. In 75% of cases, this artery originates on the left side of the aorta between the T8 and L1 vertebral segments.

Case 12

A 56-year-old man woke up with bilateral upper limb paraesthesia and weakness (with a left-sided predominance). He is having difficulty walking.

How would you manage this patient?

Take a detailed history and examine the patient to identify the nature of the problem. One would look for typical long tract signs including positive Romberg's test, diffi-culty tandem walking, Hoffman's test, clonus, upgoing plantars, brisk reflexes. One could use one of the myelopathy scores such as Nurick, Ranawat, JOA. The sudden nature of his symptoms might point to a vascular event. However, degenerative prob-lems in the spine may also present acutely.

How would you investigate him?

Investigations include bedside tests (including BP, urinary dipstick and blood glucose measurement) and radiological imaging (Cervical MRI and CT scan, Figures 4.20 and 4.21).

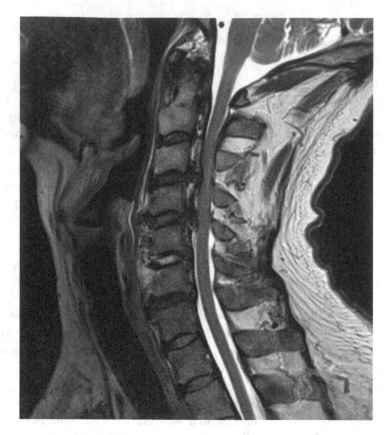

Figure 4.20 Cervical MRI scan (Case 12).

Please describe the spinal MRI scan. All the other tests were normal, including a CT head scan.

Sagittal T2-weighted spinal MRI demonstrates a multi-level disc osteophyte complex with significant spinal cord compression and signal change within the spinal cord.

What would be the next useful investigation?

Cervical CT scan.

Following are the cervical CT images. What is the diagnosis (Figure 4.21)?

Ossification of posterior longitudinal ligament (OPLL).

How would you manage this condition?

The preferred operation would be a posterior cervical decompression; however, because of the loss of cervical lordosis, this may not be effective. Moreover, an anterior cervical decompression could be considered. In addition, a C3/4 corpectomy (e.g. the worst affected level) is an alternative option. A corpectomy may be difficult because the patient is overweight and may have a short neck.

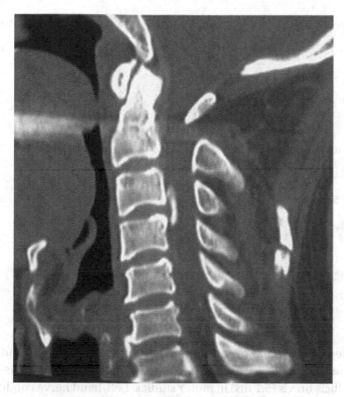

Figure 4.21 Cervical CT scan (Case 12).

Case 13

A 60-year-old woman attends a clinic with right thumb and index finger pain and paraesthesia for 9 months. Symptoms are worse at night, and she sometimes wakes up with the pain. Using the hand, for example doing up buttons can be difficult. MRI cervical spine shows no significant abnormalities.

What is the investigation shown? Please explain the findings.

Motor nerve/sites	Muscle	Latency	Amplitude	Velocity
		ms	mV	m/s
Normal values		<4.2 at wrist	>6	>50
R Median – APB				
Wrist	Abductor pollicis brevis	5.1	8.7	
Elbow	Abductor pollicis brevis	10	7.9	50
L Median – APB				
Wrist	Abductor pollicis brevis	3.4	8.2	
Elbow	Abductor pollicis brevis	8.2	7.8	51

Sensory serve/sites	Latency	Amplitude	Velocity
	ms	µV	m/s
Normal digit 2 values	<3.0	>8	>50
Right Median (digit 2)			
Wrist	Absent	Absent	Absent
Left median (digit 2)			
Wrist	2.4	12	52
Normal digit 5 values	<3.0	>6	>50
Left Ulnar (digit 5)			
Wrist	2.5	11	53
Left ulnar (digit 5)			
Wrist	2.5	9	54

These are median and ulnar nerve conduction studies. In the right hand, they show an absent median sensory response with a prolonged distal motor latency to right abductor pollicis brevis (5.1 ms) in motor studies. Left-hand nerve conduction studies are normal with normal sensory and motor amplitudes and velocities. Ulnar sensory nerve conduction studies are normal in both arms.

What is the likely diagnosis?
Carpal tunnel syndrome in the right hand. Whilst this is a clinical diagnosis, both the history and nerve conduction studies are supportive of this. The neurophysiology suggests that this is severe.

What are the typical nerve conduction findings in ulnar neuropathy at the elbow?
Sensory responses from digit 5 (little finger) are small or absent, and there is focal conduction slowing at the elbow in ulnar motor nerve conduction studies. In severe cases, motor responses are of small amplitude or absent.

Neurophysiological assessment of carpal tunnel syndrome

Specific protocols vary from laboratory to laboratory. Typically, the protocol will involve assessment of the median and ulnar sensory nerves and median motor responses as a minimum.

Sensory nerve conduction studies

One method to assess the median sensory nerve is to stimulate the index finger using ring electrodes (see Figure 4.22, left) and to record the median nerve over the wrist.

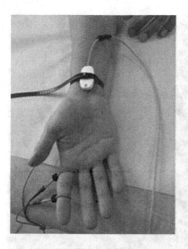
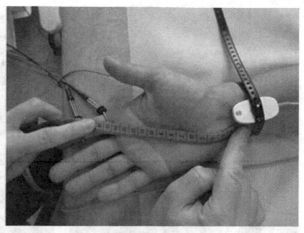

Figure 4.22 Sensory nerve conduction set-up.

The distance between the stimulating and recording electrodes is then measured to calculate a conduction velocity. The purple wire seen near the thumb is a ground electrode.

Motor nerve conduction studies

To assess motor responses, the median nerve is stimulated over the distal wrist with the recording electrodes over abductor pollicis brevis (Figure 4.22, left). The median nerve is then stimulated at the elbow (Figure 4.23, centre), and the distance between the elbow and wrist is measured (Figure 4.23, right) to obtain a forearm conduction velocity. The time from stimulation at the wrist to the initial response is the distal motor latency, and this includes the time of distal median nerve conduction, neuro-muscular junction transmission and muscle depolarization.

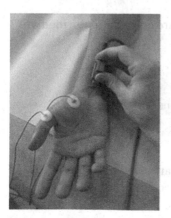
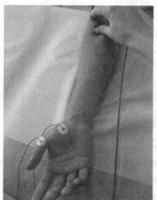
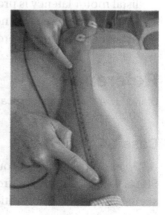

Figure 4.23 Motor nerve conduction set-up.

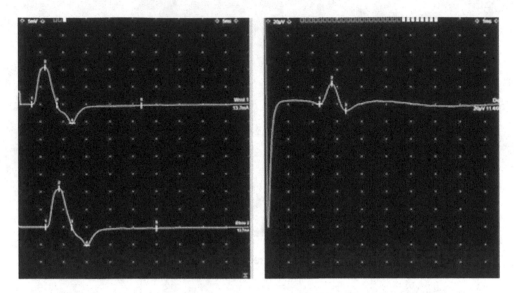

Figure 4.24 An example of normal median nerve responses. The left image is of the motor responses with the top response obtained whilst stimulating at the wrist and the bottom at the elbow. The elbow response occurs slightly later (time is on the *x*-axis and amplitude on the *y*-axis). The right image shows a normal median sensory response.

Normal values vary in different laboratories, but typically normal conduction velocities in the arms are >50 m/s and a normal distal motor latency to abductor pollicis brevis is <4.2 ms (Figure 4.24).

Neurophysiological grading of carpal tunnel syndrome

- *Mild*: Median sensory nerve conduction velocities are slow and median motor studies are normal.
- *Moderate*: Median sensory nerve conduction velocities are slow and the median distal motor latency is prolonged.
- *Severe*: Median sensory nerve conduction responses are absent and the median distal motor latency is prolonged.

Reference

Bland, J. A neurophysiological grading scale for carpal tunnel syndrome. *Muscle Nerve*. 2000; *23(8)*:1280–1283.

Case 14

A 75-year-old woman is brought into the emergency department at 23:00 after a RTA. She is GCS 15 with no neurological deficits. She was placed on a spinal board at the scene with full immobilization (Figures 4.25).

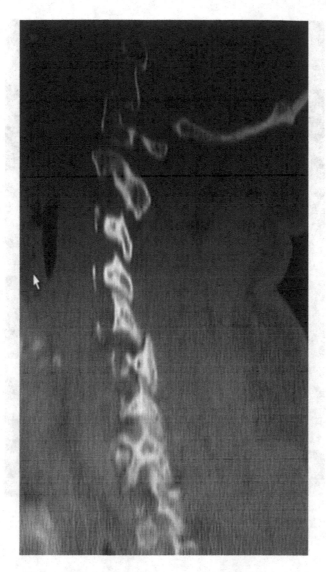

Figure 4.25 Cervical CT scan – axial slice (Case 14).

What does the scan show?

Unilateral C5/6 locked facet. The risk of neurological compromise in bilateral locked facet is very high, although there are intact patients in rare circumstances. If the degree of subluxation exceeds 50%, then it is most probably a bilateral locked facet (Figures 4.25 and 4.26).

Would you request an MRI scan at this stage?

Yes. A traumatic disc and haemorrhage should be ruled out. It is also helpful to know the integrity of spinal ligaments, particularly the posterior longitudinal ligaments (STIR sequence).

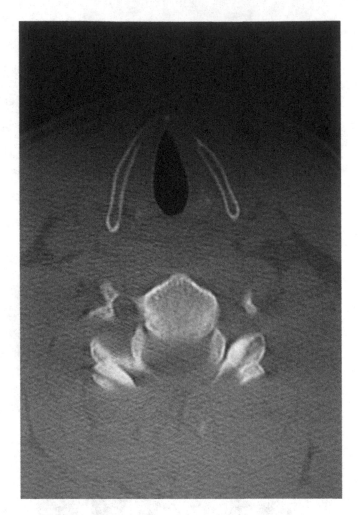

Figure 4.26 Cervical CT scan – axial slice (Case 14).

The patient starts to develop quadriparesis to MRC grade 3/5 in upper and lower limbs. What has occurred?
This would be in keeping with cord compression due to instability, traumatic disc, haematoma or progressive oedema.

How would an MRI help in surgical planning? Briefly describe the treatment options.
An MRI scan is essential to direct appropriate treatment. If one is to consider traction, it is important to assess for a cervical disc protrusion. In addition, an MRI cannot be performed after its application. Management depends on both the underlying cause of rapidly progressive quadriparesis and the patient's fitness for surgery. There are different algorithms for each scenario. If there has been a listhesis causing cord compression, correcting the slip is the priority. This may be done quickly with Gardener Wells traction and subsequent stabilization. If there is a traumatic disc prolapse, this

needs to be removed urgently. Once the discectomy has been completed, one will need to reduce the perched facet with manual traction under image intensification and place a cage and anterior plate. One could also consider a posterior fixation if thought necessary. If a reduction is not possible, the patient will need to be turned prone, the perched facet drilled and reduced, lateral mass screws placed and then turned supine again to fix anteriorly.

Halo frames still have a role but are cumbersome and have particular difficulties in the elderly or uncompliant patient. The adequacy of stability they afford is also variable.

While waiting in the MRI department, the patient develops a headache and progressive drop in consciousness. How would you investigate this?

The management would still follow the advanced trauma life support (ATLS) principles of Airway Maintenance and Cervical Spine Protection, Breathing and Ventilation, Circulation and Haemorrhage Control Disability and Exposure. This should be followed by a detailed examination to identify a localizing sign such as pupillary changes or hemiparesis. Then, the subsequent management would depend on the cause. The possibilities include the following:

1. In the trauma setting, spinal injury and an associated head injury occur in about 20% of patients. Nowadays, most significant traumas have a Camp Bastion protocol full body CT scan. However, there is a possibility that this patient did not undergo an initial head CT scan. Expanding intracranial haematoma, particularly extradural haematoma, can be missed as a result of the lucid interval. Other lesions include a subdural haematoma, contusion and associated seizure.
2. Medical causes need to be taken into account. This includes diabetes mellitus (risk of hypoglycaemia), use of drugs and substances (overdosage or withdrawal), alcoholism (withdrawal, seizures) and overdose of opiates.
3. The risk of vertebral artery dissection should be considered in patients with spinal injury that involves the foramen transversarium. The patient could develop cerebellar or brainstem infarction and oedema of the posterior fossa structures. This may even result in an acute obstructive hydrocephalus. The patient would typically present with severe headache and reducing the level of consciousness.
4. Progressive spinal cord compression at this stage as a result of instability, and this could potentially result in neurogenic shock and altered sensorium. Reassessment of her limb function and anal tone is important at this stage. In males, priapism can be seen. This can also develop iatrogenically during transfer or turning without adequate cervical spine immobilization. Other possibilities are expanding haematoma with the spinal canal, traumatic intervertebral disc and spinal artery compression.
5. Hypovolaemic shock could present in altered sensorium and be misleading. An abdominal examination and Focussed Assessment with Sonography in Trauma (FAST) would rapidly assess for gross intra-abdominal bleeding. However, guided by the patient's haemodynamic status, a chest, abdomen and pelvis CT scan should be requested if there is a suggestion of solid organ injury and evidence of haemorrhage.

If the patient initially presented with complete non-sacral-sparing paraplegia, how would you manage her?
Although the chances of good outcomes are much less in ASIA A category patients, in general, management is quite similar. Early critical care input is necessary due to the risk of ascending paresis, involvement of respiratory function and management of hypotension from neurogenic shock. From the outset, there should be careful skin care to avoid pressure sores. Similar investigation is required. Appropriate surgical stabilization will promote early mobilization out of bed. Careful counselling of the patient and their family will be vital. Early input from local spinal injury rehabilitation teams is necessary.

Case 15

A 33-year-old man is scheduled for a left subarachnoid haemorrhage. A DSA was performed for an amytal test.

What is an amytal (Wada) test and what does it assess?
A Wada test involves infusion of amytal sodium to create a temporary chemical dysfunction of either hemisphere. It is usually performed as a pre-operative investigation for lateralizing speech and memory in temporal lobe resection for epilepsy. Wada is not an acronym. It is named after the Japanese–Canadian neurologist who pioneered it.

What is the abnormality shown, and is it safe to continue with the amytal test? What precaution needs to be taken?
The angiogram shows a carotid DSA. There is an abnormal communication between the ICA and basilar artery before the carotid siphon. This could be a persistent trigeminal artery. Amytal testing would be risky in this patient because this could cause temporary dysfunction of the brainstem and cardiorespiratory arrest. However, amytal injected distal to the artery would be safe (Figure 4.27).

What adjuncts could be done to investigate a patient going for temporal lobe resection in epilepsy surgery?
Functional MRI scan and neuropsychological assessment.

Investigations revealed that he has bilateral mesial temporal lobe epilepsy (MTLE) and is not a suitable candidate for surgical resection. How would you manage him?
Discuss the patient with the epileptologist in regard to medical management. Alternatively, a vagal nerve stimulator could be offered.

Case 16

A 29-year-old woman presented via an ophthalmologist with a 3-month history of increasing headache, left facial numbness, diplopia and papilloedema. She undergoes an MRI scan (Figures 4.28–4.30).

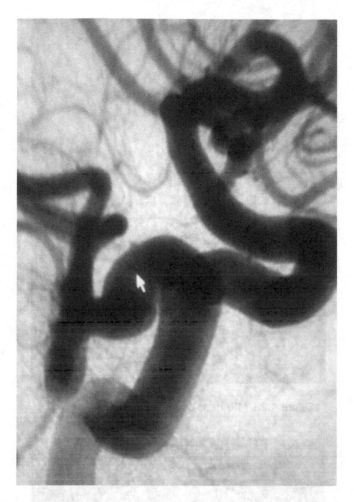

Figure 4.27 Cerebral angiogram (Case 15) (With kind permission of Dr Rufus Corkill, Consultant Radiologist, John Radcliffe Hospital, Oxford.)

How would you manage this patient?

This MRI head scan demonstrates a very large extra-axial avidly enhancing mass straddling and arising from the right sphenoid ridge. There is associated mass effect, signal change and subfalcine herniation.

The patient should be commenced on dexamethasone and a proton pump inhibitor.

The feasibility of surgical resection needs to be considered, in particular the relationship to vascular structures. Vascular imaging with CTA or MRA scans would be important. Some might consider pre-operative embolization.

What are your differential diagnoses?

- Large sphenoid wing meningioma.
- Hemangiopericytoma.
- Solitary metastatic tumour.

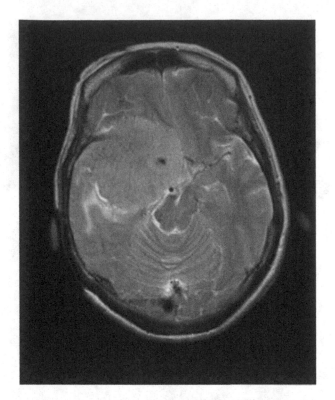

Figure 4.28 MRI Head scan – axial slice (Case 16).

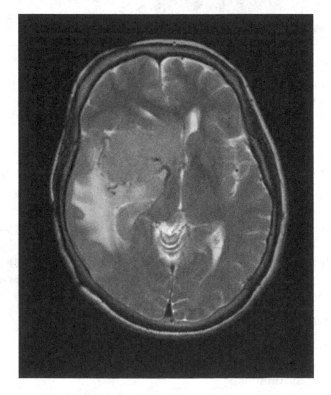

Figure 4.29 MRI Head scan – axial slice (Case 16).

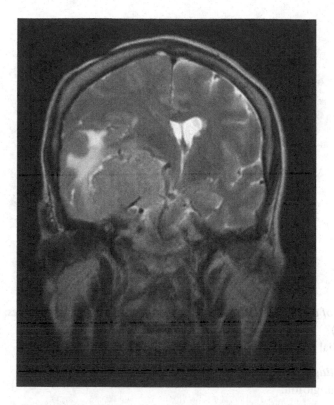

Figure 4.30 MRI Head scan – coronal slice (Case 16).

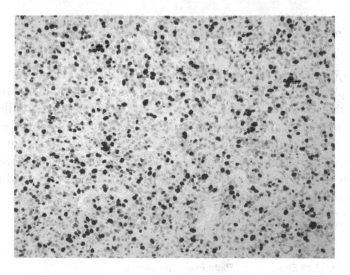

Figure 4.31 Histology slide-Ki-67 labelled (Case 16).

She went on to have resection of the tumour. What does the following slide demonstrate (Figure 4.31)?

This is a Ki-67 stained slide showing a moderately high proliferative index.

Ki-67 is a cellular marker for proliferation. It is strictly associated with cell proliferation. Ki-67 protein is present during all active phases of the cell cycle (G_1, S, G_2 and mitosis) but is absent from resting cells (G_0).

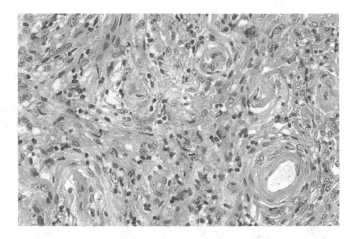

Figure 4.32 Histology slide (Case 16).

Small areas of the tumour show the following characteristic features. What is this (Figure 4.32)?
Meningothelial whorl pattern in an underlying meningioma.

What is the diagnosis?
Atypical meningioma.

Case 17

What is the investigation shown in Figure 4.33?
The picture on the left is a plot from a Humphrey visual field analyzer.

How is it performed and how does it differ from Goldmann perimetry?
The patient places their chin on a chin rest, and one eye is shielded. The patient is asked to fix their gaze on a central point. A series of white light stimuli of varying intensities is projected, and the patient must press a button when they see them. It is an automated test. Goldmann perimetry is an older technique and is not automated. In a similar way, the patient puts their chin on a chin rest covering one eye. They look into a hollow white spherical bowl. A stimulus is moved from beyond the field of vision into the field. The patient alerts the examiner when they can see the stimulus. A graphical representation is made on paper (like a dart board).

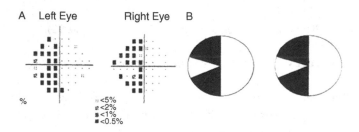

Figure 4.33 Humphrey visual fields.

What deficit does the patient have?

There is a partial left homonymous hemianopia.

Where is the lesion?

There is a disruption to the visual pathway distal to the optic tract on the right side. (This is actually typical of a lesion of the right thalamus – lateral geniculate nucleus.)

What is optic coherence tomography (OCT)?

This is an objective measurement of optic nerve fibre thickness in the optic disc of the retina. It has value in the follow-up of incidental suprasellar and peri-visual apparatus lesions and hence can dictate intervention and provide prognostication.

The Viva: The Non-operative Clinical Practice of Neurosurgery

In the UK exam, this section of the Viva covers topics not directly related to operative surgery or investigations. The spectrum of questions is therefore very wide. Although questions are generally put into a clinical context, the examiners explore a candidate's understanding of basic principles. These principles include *neurophysiology, pathophysiology, critical care, pharmacology, endocrinology, genetics, ethics and the law, research methodology, statistics, evidence base and key publications* and *standards of care.*

Many candidates spend an enormous effort memorizing precise values, ranges and units. Although specific figures are important, the emphasis of this section of the examination is to demonstrate your understanding of the basic principles.

For example: 'A positron emission tomography (PET) scan is a nuclear medical imaging technique that produces three-dimensional images. The technique involves the administration of a metabolically active, radioactive tracer that spontaneously decays to release positrons. These positrons travel a short distance into adjacent tissue where they are annihilated by reacting with electrons. This annihilation reaction results in the release of paired, high-energy photons that travel in opposite directions from each other and are detected by a PET scanner. PET imaging has potential benefits in neuro-oncology, ischaemic cerebrovascular disease and epilepsy. Limitations of this test include availability and the short half-life of isotopes. For example, the test may be challenging in the evaluation of an ictal foci in epilepsy. In these cases, a single-photon emission computed tomography (SPECT) scan is more sensitive.'

Apply your basic knowledge to real solutions. Occasionally, you may be asked to talk about a broad topic (however, most examiners would tend to avoid this). In this overwhelming situation, do not rush to mention a specific point because this may generate questions regarding only an isolated point which will lead to an incomplete answer. It is best to give a 'frame' or subdivision to the topic and then proceed to describe each point. It is recommended to begin the discussion around the most relevant or common topic.

DOI: 10.1201/9781003254379-5

Top tip: '**Define, Classify, Amplify**'

For example, if the examiner asks you to discuss the principles of 'neuroprotection', it is not advised to start with one potential treatment: hypothermia. You would then be expected to know that hypothermia results in a reduction in cerebral metabolism ($CMRO_2$) by approximately 7% per 1°C. This also leads to less oxygen and glucose consumption.

The authors recommend the following structured answer:

Define: 'Neuroprotection' refers to the preservation of neuronal structure and function by various interventions. Neuroprotection aims to prevent or slow disease progression and secondary injuries by halting or at least slowing neuronal damage.

Classify: Common mechanisms of neuronal damage include increased levels of oxidative stress, mitochondrial dysfunction, excitotoxicity, inflammatory changes, iron accumulation and protein aggregation. Common neuro-protective treatments include glutamate antagonists and antioxidants, which aim to limit excitotoxicity and oxidative stress, respectively.

Amplify: Other treatments include caspase inhibitors, trophic factors, anti-protein aggregation agents and hypothermia.

The following key topics are discussed:

1. Neuro-critical care: Management of raised intracranial pressure (ICP).
2. Seizures.
3. Hyponatraemia.
4. Diabetes insipidus (DI).
5. Brainstem testing.
6. Back pain and cauda equina syndrome.
7. Pain pathways.
8. Neuropharmacology.
9. Informed consent.
10. Management of common neurosurgical conditions.

These key topics are not a comprehensive list. The examiners will examine your logical arguments regarding controversial points. Samples of these debates are mentioned at the end of each topic (e.g. evidence of outcome measures for ICP monitoring, the overlap between syndrome of inappropriate antidiuretic hormone secretion [SIADH] and cerebral salt wasting [CSW], and screening for aneurysms).

Case scenarios

Case 1: Neuro-critical care – Management of raised intracranial pressure

An 18-year-old man is involved in a high-speed traffic accident. At the scene, his Glasgow Coma Score (GCS) is 6 (E1V1M4). On arrival at the trauma centre, he is intubated and a computed tomography (CT) scan is performed. He has diffuse cerebral oedema with effacement of the sulci. He is being monitored in the Surgical Intensive Care Unit.

How do you assess for adequate blood supply to the brain?

- **Cerebral blood flow (CBF)**: blood supply per unit area of cerebral tissue per unit time.
- Directly proportional to the volume of blood but inversely related to vascular resistance.
- CBF = cerebral perfusion pressure (CPP)/cerebral vascular resistance (CVR).
  - **Normal**: 55–60 mL per 100 g per minute.
  - **Hyperaemia**: CBF in excess of 55–60 mL per 100 g per minute.
  - **Ischaemia**: CBF below 18–20 mL per 100 g per minute.
  - **Tissue death**: CBF below 8–10 mL per 100 g per minute.

How do you control cerebral blood flow?

- Modulate factors affecting the CPP (CPP = mean arterial pressure [MAP] – ICP).
- Modulate factors affecting CVR.

CVR is controlled by four major mechanisms:

1. Metabolic control.
2. Pressure autoregulation.
3. Chemical control (by arterial pCO_2 and pO_2).
4. Neural control.

What is autoregulation? Describe the mechanisms.

- Autoregulation is the intrinsic ability of brain vasculature to maintain constant CBF over a wide range of blood pressures.
- Vessel calibre changes are mediated by an interplay between myogenic and metabolic mechanisms.
- Autoregulation can be modulated by the following:
  - Sympathetic nervous activity.
  - Renin–angiotensin system.
  - Arterial carbon dioxide tension.

What is ICP?

ICP is the pressure exerted by the intracranial contents. The Monro–Kellie hypothesis states that the sum of the intracranial volumes of blood (CBV), brain, cerebrospinal fluid (CSF), is constant, and that any additional volume increase (e.g. tumour, haematoma) must be offset by an equal decrease in another component, or else the overall pressure will rise. These volumes are contained in a rigidly fixed skull. The pressure is distributed evenly throughout the intracranial cavity (Figure 5.1).

What is a normal ICP waveform?

Normal ICP waves usually consist of three arterial components superimposed on the respiratory rhythm (Figure 5.2).

- **Percussion wave**: Arterial pressure transmitted from the choroid plexus.
- **Tidal wave:** Ventricular relaxation.
- **Dicrotic wave**: Closure of aortic valve.
- **Compliance**: dV/dP (Figure 5.3).

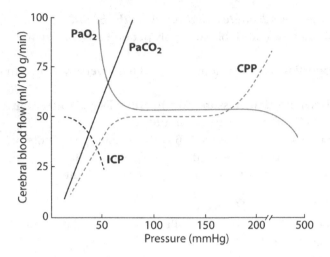

Figure 5.1 Cerebral blood flow.

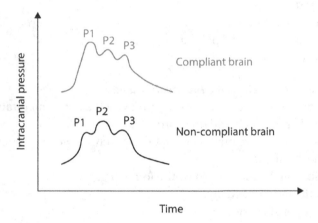

Figure 5.2 Intracranial pressure waveform.

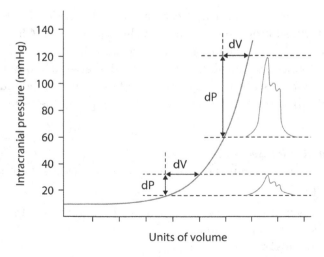

Figure 5.3 Intracranial volume pressure curve.

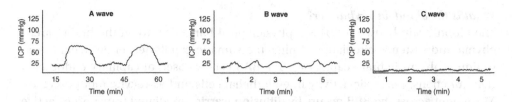

Figure 5.4 Lundberg waves. (From Elwishi M, Dinsmore J. *BJA* 2018; *19(2)*:54–59.)

What are pathological ICP waveforms?

Lundberg A waves (plateau waves)

- These indicate an abrupt increase in ICP ≥ 50 mmHg for 5–20 minutes followed by a rapid fall in ICP.
- The plateau wave represents a transient increased CBV, possibly secondary to CO_2 retention.

Lundberg B waves (pressure pulses)

- Amplitude of 10–20 mmHg with rhythmic variation 0.5–2 minutes.

Lundberg C waves

- Frequency of 4–8/minutes. Low-amplitude C wave may be seen in a normal ICP waveform. High-amplitude C wave may be pre-terminal and may sometimes be seen on top of plateau waves (Figure 5.4).

How do you manage increased ICP in a head injury patient?

1. Advanced trauma life support (ATLS)
   - ABCDE (Airway maintenance and cervical spine protection, breathing and ventilation, circulation with haemorrhage control, disability and exposure and environmental control).
2. Physiological
   - Elevate the head (30–40°); this will help reduce venous congestion.
   - Relieve jugular compression by straightening the neck and loosening bandages.
   - Avoid hypoxia and hypercarbia.
   - Maintain MAP >90 mmHg.
   - Correct electrolyte balance (hyponatraemia, hyperglycaemia).
3. Control seizures with anticonvulsants.
4. Pharmacological
   - Intubation, ventilation and sedation.
   - Adequate analgesia.
   - Osmotic diuretics: Mannitol.
   - Barbiturates may be required to obtain burst suppression on electroencephalography (EEG).
5. Surgical
   - CSF drainage procedure (external ventricular drain [EVD]).
   - Removal of causes of increased ICP (space-occupying lesion [SOL]).
   - Decompressive craniectomy.

What is the blood–brain barrier?

The blood–brain barrier (BBB) is a physiological barrier between the brain paren-chyma and systemic circulation. Unlike the somatic capillaries, endothelial fenes-tration is absent in brain capillaries. The BBB is composed of capillary endothelial tight junctions, pinocytic activity in endothelial cells and astrocytic foot processes. Movement across the BBB occurs by diffusion, carrier-mediated transport or active transport. The BBB is absent in the following areas.

- Area postrema.
- Median eminence of the hypothalamus.
- Neurohypophysis.
- Organum vasculosum (lamina terminalis).
- Pineal gland.
- Subcommissural organ.
- Subfornical organ.

The permeability across the BBB differs.

- **Highly permeable**: Water, CO_2, O_2, lipid soluble (ethanol, barbiturates).
- **Slightly permeable**: Ions (sodium, potassium and chloride).
- **Impermeable**: Plasma proteins, protein-bound molecules, large organic molecules and L-glucose.

What are the four types of cerebral oedema? Which one is associated with severe head injuries?

1. **Vasogenic:** The BBB is disrupted. Protein leaks out of the vascular system and the extracellular space expands. Plasma content leakages into the intracellular space. Vasogenic oedema responses to corticosteroids (dexamethasone). Examples include brain tumour, infection and trauma.
2. **Osmotic:** Plasma dilution decreases serum osmolality, resulting in a higher osmolality in the brain compared to the serum. This creates an abnormal pressure gradient and movement of water into the brain, which can cause swelling. Examples include hyponatraemia and SIADH.
3. **Interstitial:** There is a rupture of the CSF–brain barrier. This results in trans-ependymal flow of CSF, causing CSF to penetrate the brain and spread to the extracellular spaces and the white matter. Example includes obstructive hydrocephalus.
4. **Cytotoxic:** The BBB remains intact. There is a disruption in cellular metabolism that impairs the functioning of the sodium and potassium pump in the glial cell membrane, leading to cellular retention of sodium and water. Swollen astrocytes occur in grey and white matter. Examples include ischaemia and severe head injury.

Potential debates for discussion

Does ICP monitoring influence outcome in head injuries?
Does ICP management influence outcomes of head injuries – Evidence for decompressive craniectomy?
ICP management in paediatric head injuries.
Overlap and differentiation between the different types of brain oedema.

Case 2: Seizures

A 52-year-old woman presents with a history of chronic right-sided headaches associated with olfactory aura. Her MRI scan demonstrates a right-sided sphenoid wing meningioma.

What are seizures?

Seizures are abnormal paroxysmal cerebral neuronal discharges resulting in psychomotor and sensory abnormalities. They can be classified based on whether the source of the seizure within the brain is localized (partial) or distributed (generalized).

Partial seizures: One hemisphere involved at the onset.

1. Simple partial seizures
   - Motor.
   - Sensory.
2. Complex partial.
3. Complex partial with secondary generalization.

Generalized seizures: Bilaterally symmetrical and synchronous involving both hemispheres at the onset (with no local onset) and associated with a documented loss of conscience.

1. Absence
2. Tonic
3. Clonic
4. Generalized tonic clonic (GTC)
5. Atonic
6. Myoclonic

How do you classify seizures?

- **Symptomatic**: Seizures of known aetiology (cerebrovascular accident [CVA], trauma, tumour, vascular causes, metabolic causes or infection).
- **Idiopathic**: No underlying cause identified (juvenile myoclonic epilepsy).
- **Cryptogenic**: Seizures presumed to be symptomatic, but with unknown aetiology (West syndrome, Lennox–Gastaut syndrome).
- **Special syndromes**: Situational-related seizures (febrile seizures, alcohol withdrawal).

How do you investigate seizures?

- History and examination: It is vitally important to rule out the above-mentioned causes). Witnesses may be able to help describe the semiology of the seizure.
- Standard blood tests.
- EEG.
- Head MRI scan.

How do you manage seizures?

- Remove any reversible causes.
- Avoid factors that lower seizure threshold (e.g. sleep deprivation, hyperventilation, photic stimulation, infection, electrolyte disturbance, head injury, and cerebral ischaemia).

In general, Levetiracetam (Keppra) is the anticonvulsant of choice.

The UK National Institute for Health and Care Excellence (NICE) Guidelines (CG137 amended 2021) recommend the following.

- Newly diagnosed generalized tonic clonic seizures
  - First-line treatment in adult patients with newly diagnosed GTC seizures includes the following:
    - Sodium valproate (unless female of childbearing age)
    - Lamotrigine – if sodium valproate is unsuitable.
  - Adjunctive treatment in a patient with GTC seizures includes the following:
    - Clobazam, lamotrigine, levetiracetam, sodium valproate or topiramate if first-line treatments are ineffective or not tolerated.
  - In the presence of absence or myoclonic seizures, or if juvenile myoclonic epilepsy (JME) is suspected, do not give carbamazepine, gabapentin, oxcarbazepine, phenytoin, pregabalin, tiagabine or vigabatrin.
- Focal seizures
  - First-line treatment in a patient with newly diagnosed focal seizures includes the following:
    - Carbamazepine (unless female of childbearing age) or lamotrigine
    - Levetiracetam, oxcarbazepine or sodium valproate (teratogenic risks) – If carbamazepine and lamotrigine are unsuitable or not tolerated.
  - If the first antiepileptic drug (AED) tried is ineffective, offer an alternative from these five AEDs. Adjunctive treatment should be considered if a second well-tolerated AED is ineffective.
  - Adjunctive treatment in a patient with refractory focal seizures includes the following:
    - Carbamazepine, clobazam, gabapentin, lamotrigine, levetiracetam oxcarbazepine, sodium valproate or topiramate as adjunctive treatment in a patient with focal seizures if firstline treatments are ineffective or not tolerated.
- Petit mal or absence seizures: Treatment with ethosuximide, lamotrigine or sodium valproate.

- Myoclonic seizures: Sodium valproate.
- Infantile spasms: Vigabatrin.

Regarding the newer AEDs, NICE recommends that newer AEDs, gabapentin, lamotrigine, levetiracetam, oxcarbazepine, tiagabine, topiramate and vigabatrin, within their licensed indications, are recommended for the management of adult epilepsy who have not benefited from treatment with the older AEDs such as carbamazepine or sodium valproate, or for whom the older AEDs are unsuitable. Reasons for unsuitability include the following:

- There are contraindications to the drugs.
- They could interact with other medication (notably oral contraceptives).
- They are already known to be poorly tolerated by the individual.
- The person is a woman of childbearing potential.

Which anticonvulsants are recommended in pregnancy?

Anticonvulsant treatment is individualized. There is no one answer for this question. NICE guidelines recommend the following.

Aim for seizure freedom before conception and during pregnancy (particularly for women and girls with generalized tonic–clonic seizures). Consider the risk of adverse effects of AEDs, use the lowest effective dose of each AED, and avoid polytherapy if possible.

The clinician should discuss with the woman and girl the relative benefits and risks of adjusting medication to enable her to make an informed decision. Where appropriate, a neurologist should be consulted.

Reference

National Clinical Guideline Centre (NCGC). *The epilepsies: the diagnosis and management of the epilepsies in adults and children in primary and secondary care.* 2012 including amendments until 2021. Commissioned by the National Institute for Health and Clinical Excellence. (Please refer to your National Guidelines because they are subject to change.)

Potential debates for discussion

- Identification of pseudoseizures.
- Definition of status epilepticus and its management.
- Monitoring for seizure activity in the ventilated patient.

Case 3: Hyponatraemia

An 83-year-old woman underwent a burr-hole evacuation of a chronic subdural haematoma. On day 3, she became confused and agitated. She is diagnosed with hyponatraemia with a serum sodium of 121 mEq/L. The trend demonstrates progressive hyponatraemia.

Management of syndrome of inappropriate antidiuretic hormone secretion (SIADH)/cerebral salt-wasting syndrome (CSW).

What are the causes of hyponatraemia?
- **Hypovolaemic hyponatraemia**: Associated with low plasma volume.
  - CSW: Severe head injury, aneurysmal subarachnoid haemorrhage (SAH), and subdural haematoma.
  - Gastrointestinal loss: Vomiting and diarrhoea.
  - Excessive sweating.
  - Third space pooling: Peritonitis, pancreatitis, burns.
  - Renal insufficiency.
  - Prolonged exercise in a hot environment.
- **Euvolemic hyponatraemia**: Normal sodium stores and total body excess free water.
  - Psychogenic polydipsia.
  - Hypotonic intravenous or irrigation fluids.
- **Hypervolaemic hyponatraemia**: Inappropriate increase in sodium stores.
  - SIADH.
  - Medication (thiazide diuretics, carbamazepine, acetazolamide, angiotensin-converting enzyme inhibitors, gabapentin, haloperidol, heparin, loop diuretics, nimodipine, proton pump inhibitors, selective serotonin reuptake inhibitors).
  - Lung pathologies (e.g. pulmonary malignancy, severe COPS, acute respiratory failure, and pneumonia).
  - Hepatic cirrhosis.
  - Congestive heart failure.
  - Nephrotic syndrome.
  - Hypothyroidism.
- Cortisol deficiency.

How would you investigate this patient's hyponatraemia?
- Take a comprehensive history and examine the patient.
- Review fluid balance charts.
- Order blood test (serum and urine sodium and osmolalities, urine specific gravity, serum electrolytes, thyroid function and adrenal function).

How do you make the diagnosis of SIADH?
The diagnosis is based on history, clinical examination and blood and urine results. The patient may present with confusion, lethargy, nausea, vomiting, seizures, coma and possible fluid overload. The diagnostic criteria include hyponatraemia, inappropriately concentrated urine and evidence of renal and adrenal dysfunction.

1. Low serum sodium: <134 mEq/L.
2. Low serum osmolality: <280 mOsm/L.
3. High urinary sodium: >18 mEq/L, often 50–150.
4. High ratio of urine:serum osmolality: 1.5–2.1:1.
5. Normal renal and adrenal function.
6. No hypothyroidism.
7. No clinical signs of dehydration or overhydration.

How do you treat SIADH?

- Liaise with endocrinology.
- If mild and asymptomatic, consider fluid restriction <1 L/day (may be challenging in the cases of following a SAH).
- If severe or symptomatic, consider hypertonic saline.
- Correct hyponatraemia slowly (no more than 8-10 mmol/L of sodium per day) to prevent central pontine myelinolysis (CPM).

Biochemical marker	SIADH	CSWS
Intravascular volume status	Normal to high	Low
Serum sodium	Low	Low
Urinary sodium level	High	Very high
Vasopressin level	High	Low
Urine output	Normal or low	High
Serum uric acid level	Low	Low
Initial fractional excretion of urate	High	High
Fractional excretion of urate after correction of hyponatraemia	Normal	High
Urinary osmolality	High	High
Serum osmolality	Low	Low
Blood urea nitrogen/creatinine level	Low to normal	High
Serum potassium level	Normal	Normal to high
Central venous pressure	Normal to high	Low
Pulmonary capillary wedge pressure	Normal to high	Low
Brain natriuretic peptide level	Normal	High
Treatment	Water restriction	Fluids and/or mineralocorticoid

CSWS = cerebral salt-wasting syndrome, SIADH = syndrome of inappropriate antidiuretic hormone.

Case 4: Management of diabetes insipidus

A 43-year-old man underwent an endoscopic endonasal resection of a craniopharyngioma. Post-operatively, the patient is thirsty with a high urine output >300 mL/hours.

What is his diagnosis?

DI is a result of low circulating levels of antidiuretic hormone (ADH) (or rarely, renal insensitivity secondary to ADH). The insufficiency of ADH results in excessive renal loss of water and electrolytes. Patients have a high output of dilute urine (<200 mOsm/L or specific gravity <1.003) with normal or high serum osmolality. They often present with a craving for fluids.

DI can be classified into central/neurogenic or nephrogenic DI.

Central/neurogenic DI is caused by hypothalamic-pituitary axis dysfunction.

- Familial (autosomal dominant).
- Idiopathic.
- Post-traumatic (including surgery).
- Tumour (craniopharyngioma, metastasis, lymphoma).
- Granuloma (neurosarcoidosis, histiocytosis).
- Infection (meningitis, encephalitis).
- Autoimmune.
- Vascular (aneurysm, Sheehan's syndrome).

Nephrogenic DI is associated with relative resistance of the kidney to normal or supranormal levels of ADH.

- Familial (X-linked recessive).
- Hypokalemia.
- Hypercalcemia.
- Sjögren's syndrome.
- Drugs: Lithium.
- Chronic renal disease.

How do you make the diagnosis?
1. Dilute urine.
   - Urine osmolality <200 mOsm/L or specific gravity <1.003.
   - Inability to concentrate urine to >300 mOsm/L in the presence of clinical dehydration.
2. Urine output >250 mL/hours.
3. Normal or above-normal serum sodium.
4. Normal adrenal function.

What is the triphasic response?
Following transsphenoidal surgery or removal of a craniopharyngioma, central DI results because of injury to the posterior pituitary. Three patterns are seen.

- **Transient DI**: Supra-normal urine output and polydipsia that normalizes within 12–36 hours.
- **Prolonged DI**: Supra-normal urine output occurs for prolonged periods of time (months to years).
- **Triphasic DI**
  - **Phase 1**: Injury to the pituitary gland reduces ADH levels for 4–5 days, and patients present with polyuria/polydipsia.
  - **Phase 2**: Cell death releases ADH for the next 4–5 days, and there is a transient normalization or even SIADH-like water retention.
  - **Phase 3**: Reduced or absent ADH secretion results in transient or prolonged DI.

How do you manage DI?
If DI is mild and the patient's thirst mechanism is intact, instruct the patient to drink only when thirsty; in this way, patients can usually keep up with their fluid losses. If DI is severe, patients may not be able to take in an adequate intake of fluids to meet

their losses. In these cases, desmopressin (DDVAP) can be given by the oral, nasal or intravenous route.

Potential debates for discussion

- The overlap between SIADH and CSW.
- Switchover phases between CSW and SIADH.
- Adipsic DI.

Case 5: Brainstem testing

A 73-year-old man is thrown off his motorbike while driving home. He lost control as a result of bad weather. On arrival at the emergency department, his GCS is 3, and his pupils are fixed and dilated.

What is brainstem death?

Brainstem death is diagnosed by the cessation of function *and* irreversibility of cessation of either the cardiopulmonary system or the entire brain.

What are the brainstem death criteria?

In the UK, the tests should be carried out by two qualified doctors who are competent with the procedure; one of them should be a consultant, and both should have been fully registered with the General Medical Council for at least 5 years. The test must be undertaken by the two doctors and completed successfully on two separate occasions.

Exclusion criteria: Reversible causes (e.g. hypothermia, drugs, metabolic and endocrine abnormalities and shock) should be corrected.

Ventilator dependence is confirmed by disconnection for a period to ensure that the medullary respiratory centre is exposed to a powerful hypercapnic drive stimulus ($PaCO_2 \geq 6.65$ kPa or >60 mmHg).

The prescribed testing is required to be repeated, at an unspecified interval, 'to ensure that there has been no observer error'.

Potential debates for discussion

Absence of brainstem reflexes	
Absent pupillary light reflex	Pupils are fixed and do not respond to light.
Absent corneal reflexes	
Absent oculovestibular reflex	In a clean and unobstructed ear canal, 20 mL of iced water is irrigated. There should be no eye movement in response to the cold stimulus.
Absent oculocephalic reflex	Sudden rotation of the head from side to side results in a negative doll's eye, in which the eyes would stay fixed in mid-orbit position.
Absent gag and cough reflex	

(Continued)

Absence of brainstem reflexes *(Continued)*	
Apnoea test	The patient is pre-oxygenated with 100% oxygen; the ventilator is turned off, and oxygen is given via nasal cannula (6–8 L/min); blood gases are obtained; when $PaCO_2$ >6.65 kPA or >60 mmHg, the apnoea test is positive if there is no respiratory effort.
No response to deep central pain	No response to supraorbital painful stimuli.
Observations	Core temperature >32.2°C, SBP ≥90 mmHg.

Role and interpretation of brainstem auditory evoked potentials (BSAEP), transcranial Doppler (TCD) and angiography in brainstem death tests.

Case 6: Back pain and cauda equina syndrome

A 32-year-old woman presents with an acute-on-chronic history of lower back pain. After returning from a ski holiday, she presents with a severe episode of back pain, bilateral lower limb weakness and urinary incontinence.

What are the 'red flags' on clinical history and examination?

Clinical history

- Age >50 years.
- Cancer: History of cancer, unexplained weight loss, pain at multiple sites.
- Night pain (not mechanical in nature).
- Immunosuppression: Human immunodeficiency virus (HIV), steroid use, diabetes mellitus (DM), organ transplantation.
- Infection: Fever, night sweats, back tenderness, limited range of movement.
- Cauda equina syndrome (CES): Sphincter dysfunction, saddle anaesthesia, leg pain, leg paraesthesia or leg weakness.
- Trauma: Major or minor (e.g. osteoporotic patients).
- Intractability.
- Neurological symptoms.

Clinical examination

- Saddle anaesthesia.
- Incontinence.
- Fever >38°C.
- Urinary retention.
- Muscular weakness.
- Bony tenderness (vertebral).
- Limited range of spinal motion.

How do you differentiate between neurogenic and vascular claudication?

Neurogenic claudication

Symptoms
- Leg pain on standing or walking.

- Weakness, 'giving way'.
- Associated with numbness (dermatomal).
- Worse with walking or standing.
- Relieved quickly with sitting or bending forward.

Signs
- Normal examination.
- The following may be present:
  - Reduced deep tendon reflexes.
  - Dermatomal paraesthesia.
  - Positive straight leg raise test.
  - Wide-based gait.

Vascular claudication

Symptoms
- Calf pain with walking.
- Buttock, thigh pain ± foot pain.
- Worse when walking or activity.
- Relieved with minutes of rest.
- Paraesthesia ± weakness.
- Rest pain (advanced).

Signs
- Reduced pulses and bruits.
- Skin changes (arterial insufficiency).
- Pallor on elevation.
- Dusky rubor on dependence (Buerger's test).

What is cauda equina syndrome?

CES is a spinal emergency in which damage to the cauda equina results in loss of function of the lumbar plexus (nerve roots) of the spinal canal below the termination (conus medullaris) of the spinal cord.

What are the most common symptoms and signs of cauda equina syndrome?

- Lower back pain.
- Bilateral sciatica.
- Saddle anaesthesia.
- Motor weakness of the lower limbs.
- Urinary dysfunction (e.g. retention and incontinence).
- Bowel dysfunction (e.g. reduced anal sphincter tone, incontinence).

Where are the bladder control centres?

There are three main centres:

- **Frontal lobe**: Anteromedial frontal lobe and corpus callosum, which are involved in conscious inhibition.
- **Nucleus locus coeruleus of the pons**: Synchronizes the detrusor muscle contraction with the relaxation of the urethral sphincter. It regulates both sympathetic and parasympathetic responses.
- **Sacral centre**: The reflex centre.

Describe the physiology of bladder control

The lower urinary tract is innervated by three principal sets of peripheral nerves involving the parasympathetic, sympathetic and somatic nervous systems from three major nerves, namely, the pelvic, hypogastric and pudendal nerves, respectively.

Motor control

Autonomic (involuntary)

- **Parasympathetic control**: S2–S4 (cell bodies in intermediolateral column of the grey matter of the spinal cord) to the pelvic splanchnic nerves (nervi erigentes) to the ganglia in the muscle wall (detrusor muscles).
- **Sympathetic control**: T12–L2 (cell bodies in intermediolateral column of the grey matter of the spinal cord) to the pre-ganglionic axons to inferior mesenteric ganglion to the inferior hypogastric plexus to the bladder wall and internal sphincters.

Somatic control (voluntary)

- Control originates from the frontal lobe and descends along the pyramidal tract into the pudendal nerve to innervate the external sphincters.

Sensory control

Bladder distension is detected by sensory stretch receptors on the muscle wall. An action potential is generated along the first-order sensory neurons, which travel along the autonomic fibres (via pelvic, hypogastric and pudendal nerves) to the conus medullaris and then ascend primarily in the spinothalamic tract.

How should this patient be managed?

The patient requires an urgent spinal operation (e.g. microdiscectomy, lumbar decompression). The timing of surgery is essential. Following surgery, input from the neuro-urologist, physiotherapists and rehabilitation should be considered.

Potential debates for discussion

- Role of spinal fixation in cases of back pain without spondylolisthesis.
- Role of discography in selecting patients for spinal fixation with 'discogenic' back pain.
- Role and importance of urodynamic studies in identifying incomplete recovery from cauda equina syndrome.

Case 7: Pain pathways

A 43-year-old man underwent an elective craniotomy to debulk an underlying SOL. Six hours after the surgery, he develops moderate headaches and sharp pain around the incision site.

What is pain and what are its mechanisms of transmission?

Pain is a physiological response to noxious stimuli (e.g. thermal, mechanical, chemical or trauma) that are damaging to the underlying tissues. Mechanisms of pain transmission are classified in the following.

- **Transduction** – The mechanism by which receptors are activated. Noxious stimulus is converted into electrochemical stimulus, which in turn is converted into an electrochemical impulse.
- **Transmission** – The mechanism by which an electrochemical impulse travels in the dorsal horn of the spinal cord to the thalamus and cortex.
- **Modulation** – The mechanism by which the pain impulse is dampened or amplified; it occurs primarily in the dorsal horn of the spinal cord.
- **Perception** – It refers to the subjective experience of pain that results from the interaction of transduction, transmission, modulation and the psychological aspects of the individual.

There are two main components of the spinothalamic tract (Figure 5.5).

1. The lateral spinothalamic tract transmits pain and temperature.
2. The anterior spinothalamic tract (or ventral spinothalamic tract) transmits crude touch and pressure.

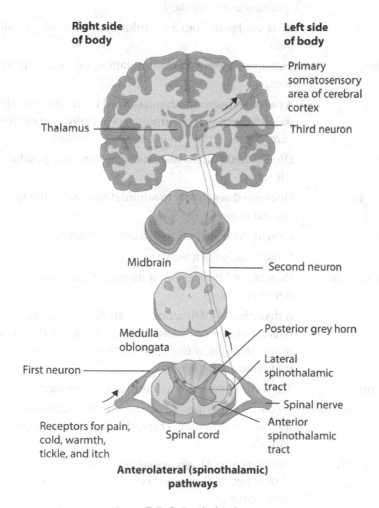

Figure 5.5 Spinothalamic tract.

The International Association for the Study of Pain (IASP) defines the following key pain terms:

Pain	An unpleasant sensory and emotional experience associated with actual or potential tissue damage or described in terms of such damage.
Allodynia	Pain due to a stimulus that does not normally provoke pain.
Analgesia	Absence of pain in response to stimulation which would normally be painful.
Anaesthesia dolorosa	Pain in an area or region that is anaesthetic.
Causalgia	A syndrome of sustained burning pain, allodynia, and hyperpathia after a traumatic nerve lesion, often combined with vasomotor and sudomotor dysfunction and later trophic changes.
Dysesthesia	An unpleasant abnormal sensation, whether spontaneous or evoked.
Hyperalgesia	Increased pain from a stimulus that normally provokes pain.
Hyperesthesia	Increased sensitivity to stimulation, excluding the special senses.
Hyperpathia	A painful syndrome characterized by an abnormally painful reaction to a stimulus, especially a repetitive stimulus, as well as an increased threshold.
Hypoalgesia	Diminished pain in response to a normally painful stimulus.
Hypoesthesia	Decreased sensitivity to stimulation, excluding the special senses.
Neuralgia	Pain in the distribution of a nerve or nerves.
Neuritis	Inflammation of a nerve or nerves.
Neuropathic pain	Pain caused by a lesion or disease of the somatosensory nervous system.
Neuropathy	A disturbance of function or pathological change in a nerve. (One nerve: mononeuropathy; several nerves: mononeuropathy multiplex; diffuse and bilateral: polyneuropathy.)
Nociception	The neural process of encoding noxious stimuli.
Nociceptive neuron	A central or peripheral neuron of the somatosensory nervous system that is capable of encoding noxious stimuli.
Nociceptive pain	Pain that arises from actual or threatened damage to non-neural tissue and is due to the activation of nociceptors.

Nociceptive stimulus	An actually or potentially tissue-damaging event transduced and encoded by nociceptors.
Nociceptor	A high-threshold sensory receptor of the peripheral somatosensory nervous system that is capable of transducing and encoding noxious stimuli.
Noxious stimulus	A stimulus that is damaging or threatens damage to normal tissues.
Pain threshold	The minimum intensity of a stimulus that is perceived as painful.
Pain tolerance level	The maximum intensity of a pain-producing stimulus that a subject is willing to accept in a given situation.
Paraesthesia	An abnormal sensation, whether spontaneous or evoked.
Sensitization	Increased responsiveness of nociceptive neurons to their normal input, and/or recruitment of a response to normally subthreshold inputs.
Central sensitization	Increased responsiveness of nociceptive neurons in the central nervous system to their normal or subthreshold afferent input.
Peripheral sensitization	Increased responsiveness and reduced threshold of nociceptive neurons in the periphery to the stimulation of their receptive fields.

What is the 'gate control' theory?

In 1965, the gate control theory was described by Melzack and Wall. The theory explains that perception of physical pain is not a direct result of activation of nociceptors but is rather modulated by an interaction between different neurons, both pain-transmitting and non-pain transmitting, in the substantia gelatinosa of the spinal cord. A gate control system modulates sensory input from the skin before it evokes pain perception and response.

- Aδ fibres are fast and myelinated (transmission occurs in 0.1 s, travels 6–30 m/s); they transmit pain as sharp and electric in nature.
- C fibres are slow and unmyelinated (transmission occurs after 1 s but increases over additional seconds to minutes, travels 0.05–2 m/s); they transmit pain as burning, aching or throbbing in nature.
- Aβ fibres are large-diameter fibres that are non-nociceptive (e.g. do not transmit pain stimuli) and inhibit the effects of Aδ and C fibres.

Large myelinated fibres have negative dorsal root potentials, and smaller C fibres have positive potentials. Stimulation of the larger fibres prevents the transmission of pain impulses in the smaller fibres by maintaining a negative potential in the dorsal horn.

Potential debates for discussion

- Utility of intrathecal morphine pumps.
- Current indications and techniques of cordotomy.
- Discussion of pain killer medication and their site of action in the nervous system
- Efficacy of occipital nerves stimulation.

Summary

Allodynia	Lowered threshold	Stimulus and response mode differ.
Hyperalgesia	Increased response	Stimulus and response mode are similar.
Hyperpathia	Raised threshold: increased response	Stimulus and response mode may be the same or different.
Hypoalgesia	Raised threshold: lowered response	Stimulus and response mode are similar.

Case 8: Neuropharmacology

Case 8A

A 31-year-old man presents to the trauma centre after sustaining a gunshot wound to the head. The patient is immediately intubated, ventilated and sedated. On examination, his GCS was 3 with equal and reactive pupils. His head CT scan demonstrates sulci effacement, diffuse subarachnoid blood and a bullet fragment in the left parietal lobe. His EEG shows seizure activity. After 1 hours, his ICP readings continue to rise up to 40 cm H_2O.

Describe the pharmacology of the following medications, which are used to treat his elevated ICP and control his seizures.

1. Mannitol

Mode of action
- An osmotic diuretic results in immediate plasma expansion. It reduces blood viscosity and haematocrit, which in turn increases CBF and O_2 delivery, and therefore improve the overall blood rheology.
- Causes include an increase in the intravascular volume by drawing water from the cerebral parenchyma.
- A free-radical scavenger.
- Supports the microcirculation.

Complications
- Opens the endothelial cells in the BBB, which can potentially aggravate vasogenic oedema.
- Hypertension.
- Hyperosmolar state leading to renal failure (e.g. acute tubular necrosis).
- Electrolyte derangement (e.g. hypernatraemia).

2. Levetiracetam

Mode of action

- Thought to be due to binding to synaptic vesicle protein 2A (SV2A). SV2A is a membrane-bound protein, which has a role in vesicle exocytosis and regulation of the amount of secretory vesicles available for neurotransmission. It has a wide therapeutic index with minimal pharmakinetc interactions.

Complications

- Headaches.
- Fatigue.
- Blocked nose.
- Itchy throat.
- Anxiety.
- Depression.

3. Phenytoin

Mode of action

- Phenytoin blocks sustained high-frequency repetitive firing of action potentials. This is accomplished by reducing the amplitude of sodium-dependent action potentials through enhancing steady-state inactivation. Sodium channels exist in three main confirmations (e.g. resting, open or inactive states). Phenytoin binds preferentially to the inactive form and blocks sodium channels.

Pharmacokinetics

- Mixed-order kinetics at therapeutic concentrations.
- First-order kinetics at low levels.
- Zero-order kinetics at high levels.

Complications

- Allergy (fever, rash, polyarthritis).
- Carcinogenesis.
- Cerebellar dysfunction and degeneration (e.g. nystagmus, ataxia).
- Cognitive dysfunction.
- Coarse facial features.
- Dermatological disorders (hypertrichosis and hirsutism).
- Diplopia.
- Gingival hypertrophy.
- Haematological disorders (low folate levels, megaloblastic anaemia).
- Hepatic granulomas.
- Hypersensitivity.
- Teratogenicity.
- Systemic lupus erythematosus (SLE)-like syndrome.
- Stevens–Johnson syndrome.
- Stupor.
- Peripheral neuropathy.

Signs of toxicity (use the mnemonic: SCAND):

- **S**lurred speech.
- **C**onfusion – CNS depression.
- **A**sterixis.

- Nystagmus.
- Diplopia.

4. Carbamazepine

Mode of action
- Carbamazepine stabilizes the inactive state of voltage-gated sodium channels and potentiates gamma-aminobutyric acid (GABA) receptors.

Pharmacokinetics
- Carbamazepine is slowly metabolized, but well absorbed after oral administration. Its plasma half-life is 20–55 hours when given as a single dose. It is a strong inducer of hepatic enzymes, and the plasma half-life shortens to ~15 hours when it is given repeatedly.

Complications
- Drowsiness and gastrointestinal upset.
- Headache and migraines, motor coordination impairment.
- SIADH.
- Relative leukopenia.
- Haematological toxicity (agranulocytosis, aplastic anaemia).
- Hepatitis.
- Stevens–Johnson syndrome.
- Transient diplopia.
- Ataxia.

Case 8B

A 76-year-old man presents with tremor, rigidity, bradykinesia and recurrent falls.

Select a medication used to treat Parkinson's disease and explain the pharmacology.

Sinemet

Sinemet (carbidopa-levodopa) is used to treat Parkinson's disease. **Carbidopa**, an inhibitor of aromatic amino acid decarboxylation, blocks the metabolism of levodopa in the liver, decreasing nausea and increasing the amount of levodopa that reaches the brain. **Levodopa**, an aromatic amino acid, is rapidly converted into dopamine by the enzyme dopa decarboxylase (DDC), which is present in the central and peripheral nervous systems. The majority of levodopa is metabolized before it reaches the brain. Levodopa is most effective in treating bradykinesia and rigidity but less effective in reducing tremor and improving gait imbalance.

Side effects include abnormal muscle movement, chorea, confusion, depression, difficulty sleeping, dry mouth, dizzy spells, hallucinations, loss of appetite, nausea, sleepiness, vomiting and weakness.

What is the surgical treatment for Parkinson's disease?

Tissue transplantation (research phase)

Tissue transplantation involves the implantation of foetal dopaminergic brain cells into Parkinson's disease patients. Other options include using the patient's own adrenal medulla.

Pallidotomy

Pallidotomy directly destroys a portion of the internal segment of the globus pallidus (GPi), interrupting pallidofugal pathways or diminishing inputs to the medial pallidum (including the subthalamic nucleus [STN]).

Electrical stimulation

Electrical stimulation consists of deep brain stimulation (DBS) to the GPi and STN. Patients are considered for DBS if they have been refractory to medical treatment and their main symptoms are rigidity or bradykinesia. If tremor is also present, consider the ventralis intermedius (VIM) target.

Case 8C

A 59-year-old woman presents with a 3-week history of deterioration in her speech and left-sided weakness. Her MRI scan demonstrates a large enhancing frontal SOL with significant oedema. She is started on dexamethasone. She undergoes a craniotomy to debulk her SOL. Formal histology confirms the diagnosis of a glioblastoma multiforme (GBM).

Describe the pharmacology of the following medications, which are used to medically address her brain swelling.

Dexamethasone

Mode of action
- Dexamethasone is a potent synthetic member of the glucocorticoid class of steroid drugs that has anti-inflammatory and immunosuppressant effects. It is 25 times more potent than cortisol in its glucocorticoid effect while having minimal mineralocorticoid effect. Glucocorticoids enter cells through passive diffusion and form a complex with a receptor protein. This complex then undergoes an irreversible activation and enters the cell nucleus, where it binds to DNA, leading to biological effects induced by these hormones, including increased hepatic gluconeogenesis, increased lipolysis, muscle catabolism, and inhibition of peripheral glucose uptake in muscle and adipose tissue. In addition, dexamethasone increases angiopoietin-1 and decreases vascular endothelial growth factor (VEGF) in the endothelial cell.

Pharmacokinetics
- Dexamethasone is metabolized by the liver. Its half-life is 1.8–3.5 hours.

Function
- Reduce peritumoural and vasogenic brain oedema.
- Reduce increased ICP.
- Decrease frequency of plateau waves.
- Decrease cerebral spinal fluid production.
- Decrease tumour cerebral blood.

Complications
- Gastrointestinal: Gastritis and steroid ulceration, pancreatitis, intestinal perforation, elevated liver enzymes, fatty liver degeneration and hiccups.
- Cardiovascular and renal: Hypertension, sodium and salt retention and hypokalemic acidosis.

- Central nervous system: Progressive multifocal leukoencephalopathy (PML), mental agitation, epidural lipomatosis and pseudotumour cerebri.
- Endocrine: Weight gain, hyperlipidaemia, Cushing's syndrome, glucose intolerance and DM.
- Ophthalmological: Posterior subcapsular cataracts and glaucoma.
- Musculoskeletal: Avascular necrosis, osteoporosis and muscle wasting.
- Haematological: Hypercoagulopathy, demargination of white blood cells – increasing the white blood cell count, immunosuppressant action (pre-disposition to bacterial, viral and fungal infections).
- Psychiatric disturbances: Depression, personality changes, irritability, euphoria mania and mood swings.
- Dermatological: Acne, allergic dermatitis, dry scaly skin, ecchymoses, petechiae, erythema, impaired wound healing, increased sweating, rash, striae, suppression of reactions to skin tests, thin fragile skin, thinning scalp hair and urticaria.

Potential debates for discussion

- Role of steroids in spinal cord injuries.
- Speed of action of steroids in tumoural brain oedema.
- Role of steroids in non-tumoural brain oedema.

Case 9: Informed consent

Case 9A

A 63-year-old man, who is unconscious, requires a life-saving emergency craniotomy to evacuate an extradural haematoma. A 7-year-old boy requires a revision of his ventriculoperitoneal (VP) shunt.

Who provides consent in these situations?

The 63-year-old man is unconscious and requires an emergency operation. In the case of an unconscious patient, the next of kin should be notified. If no next of kin is available, it is best to obtain a colleague's agreement with the surgical procedure proposed and document this in the medical notes. The law recognizes that it is in the patient's best interest to go ahead with such an emergency treatment. In the case of the 7-year-old boy who requires a revision of his VP shunt, children under the age of 16 are legally unable to give consent, and the parent or guardian should provide consent on their behalf. The procedure and its potential benefits and risks should be explained to the child, parent or guardian.

What are the principles of consent?

- Informed consent means that the procedure is carefully explained to the patient in a balanced and unemotional way, stating the benefits and the significant risks associated with the procedure. Alternative treatments must also be explained.
- The patient has a legal right to withhold consent if of sound mind.

1. **Informed consent** – The patient has adequate information to make a decision.
   - Explain why you think a proposed treatment is necessary.
   - Explain the benefits and potential risks of the proposed treatment.
   - Explain what might happen if this treatment is not carried out.
   - Explain what other forms of treatment are available with their risks and benefits.
2. **Voluntary decision** – The patient has made the decision.
3. **Ability** – The patient has the ability to weigh the benefits and risks of surgery and make an informed decision.

What about children over the age of 16?

Once children reach the age of 16, they are presumed by the law to be competent. They are able to give consent for themselves for their own medical and surgical treatment along with any associated procedures, including investigations or anaesthesia. However, it is the best practice to encourage competent children to involve their families in the decision-making process.

What is competency?

The patient comprehends, retains and weighs the information in order to make an informed decision regarding treatment.

What happens if a child aged 16 or 17 is not competent?

If a child is aged 16 or 17 and not competent to make an informed decision, then a person with parental responsibility can make the decision for them. However, the child should still be involved as much as possible in the process.

What happens when a child reaches the age of 18?

Once children reach the age of 18, no one else can make the decisions on their behalf. If an 18 year old is not competent to make their own decisions, clinicians can provide treatment, and that is in the patient's 'best interest'.

What happens to a child under the age of 16?

Children younger than 16 are not automatically presumed to be legally competent to make decisions about their healthcare. However, the courts have stated that children under the age of 16 will be competent to give valid consent to a particular intervention if they have 'sufficient understanding and intelligence to enable them to understand fully what is proposed', known as 'Gillick competence'. As with older children, you must respect requests from a competent patient under the age of 16 by keeping their treatment confidential.

Should the consent form be signed?

Legally, it makes no difference whether the patient signs a form to indicate consent or whether they give consent orally or even non-verbally (e.g. holding out an arm for their blood pressure to be taken). A consent form is only a record, not proof that genuine consent has been given. It is the best practice to seek written consent and also to document this in the patient's medical notes.

When is it lawful to provide a treatment based on the child's best interests?
- Emergency – No one with parental responsibility is available.
- Emergency – Available parents not capable of providing informed consent (e.g. under the influence of alcohol).

Case 9B

A 47-year-old singer songwriter develops a vocal cord paralysis following an anterior cervical discectomy and fusion. A 60-year-old gentleman, who presented with brainstem compression, develops a winged scapula following a resection of large vestibular schwannoma in the park bench position.

The *Montgomery vs. Lanarkshire* case of March 2015, is a landmark case that is essential knowledge for providing lawful consent in the UK. The case concerned the vaginal delivery of a child to a woman with short stature and diabetes. The child had a difficult birth due to shoulder dystocia and ended up with cerebral palsy. The courts found in the claimant's favour that she should have been told about this possible complication and should have been offered a caesarian section. Previously, the 'Bolam test' would apply (e.g. if a doctor reaches the standard of a responsible body of medical opinion, he is not negligent). This case overthrew that paternalistic approach to consent instead establishing a duty of care to warn of material risks. The test of materiality in the Montgomery case was whether 'a reasonable person in the patient's position would be likely to attach significance to the risk, or the doctor is or should reasonably be aware that the particular patient would be likely to attach significance to it'.

In the above examples, it would be quite likely that a singer song writer who developed a vocal cord palsy would win a negligence claim if the risks of the vocal cord palsy were not made clear to him pre-operatively. For the second case, a negligence claim would be much less likely to be successful. A winged scapula is unlikely to have been considered a material risk to someone undergoing a very large operation for a life-threatening problem, particularly given the rarity of the complication.

Potential debates for discussion

> Blood transfusion in paediatric cases involving Jehovah's Witness families.

Case 10: Management of common neurosurgical conditions

Case 10A

An 83-year-old woman reports right-sided facial pain in the V1 and V2 distribution. She has been diagnosed with trigeminal neuralgia.

What are the management options for this condition?
Trigeminal neuralgia can be managed by medical and surgical treatment.

- Medical treatment: Carbamazepine, gabapentin.
- Surgical treatment.

- Peripheral nerve ablation or neurectomy.
- Percutaneous trigeminal rhizotomy.
  - Chemical: Glycerol injection into Meckel's cave.
  - Electrical: Radiofrequency thermocoagulation.
  - Mechanical: Balloon compression.
- Microvascular decompression (MVD).
- Stereotactic radiosurgery.

The following factors will help in determining which treatment option is ideal for the patient:

- Age.
- Comorbidities.
- Failure of medical management.
- Patient's choice.

Potential debates for discussion

- Efficacy, limitations and targets for stereotactic radiosurgery (STRS) in trigeminal neuralgia.
- Mode of action of medications.

Case 10B

A 33-year-old woman reports headaches, visual deterioration and amenorrhea. She has been diagnosed with Cushing's disease (Figure 5.6).

What investigations should be performed for this condition?

The diagnosis of Cushing's disease should be confirmed. Obtain a detailed history and examine the cardiovascular, respiratory and neurological systems. Collaboration with an Endocrinologist is recommended. Further investigations include general and specific investigations.

General tests: Full blood count, urea and electrolytes, urine dipstick (assess for glucose: diabetes), chest radiography and ECG.

Specific tests

- Pituitary function test (e.g. prolactin, 8 a.m. cortisol, follicle-stimulating hormone [FSH], luteinizing hormone [LH], T4, thyroid-stimulating hormone [TSH], insulin-like growth factor-1 [IGF-1], fasting glucose).
- Twenty-four hour of urine-free cortisol (suggestive of hypercortisolaemia if >3× normal).
- Overnight low-dose dexamethasone suppression test (to establish a primary or secondary cause).
- Adrenocorticotrophic hormone (ACTH) levels.
- Visual field assessment.
- MRI Head scan.
- Further assessment: Synacthen test (ACTH stimulation test) assesses the functioning of the adrenal gland stress response by measuring the adrenal

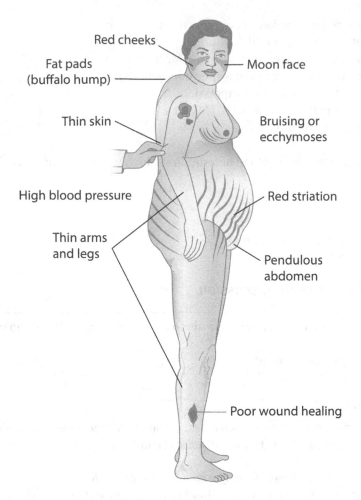

Red cheeks

Fat pads
(buffalo hump)

Moon face

Thin skin

Bruising or
ecchymoses

High blood pressure

Red striation

Thin arms
and legs

Pendulous
abdomen

Poor wound healing

Figure 5.6 Signs of Cushing's syndrome.

response to ACTH. ACTH is a hormone produced in the anterior pituitary gland
that stimulates the adrenal glands to release cortisol, dehydroepiandrosterone
(DHEAS) and aldosterone. It is a useful investigation in cases of suspected reduced
pituitary ACTH production reserve. It is used to diagnose or exclude primary and
secondary adrenalin sufficiency, Addison's disease and related conditions. In
addition to quantifying adrenal insufficiency, the test can distinguish whether the
cause is adrenal (low cortisol and aldosterone production) or pituitary (low ACTH
production).

- A synthetic analogue of ACTH, cosyntropin 0.25 mg, is administered by the
  intravenous or the intramuscular route.
- Cortisol levels are drawn before the dose is administered and again 30 minutes
  after administration.
- If the increase in cortisol is less than 6 mcg/dL, the hypothalamic–pituitary axis
  is still suppressed and the patient still requires supplementation for another
  4 weeks. If the increase is greater than 6 mcg/dL, the patient no longer requires
  steroid therapy because adrenal function has returned to normal.
- Petrosal sampling procedure: In cases of diagnostic dilemma, you can confirm the
  source of ACTH and help predict the lateralization of Cushing's disease.

Post-operative morning cortisol levels are typically measured 72 hours after surgery. In the post-operative period, morning cortisol levels are typically low because normal ACTH-producing cells in the pituitary gland have been suppressed by elevated serum cortisol levels. Therefore, the removal of the ACTH-secreting tumour leaves no source of ACTH. The adrenal glands are no longer stimulated and cortisol levels drop. It is important to note that up to 30% of patients with long-term cures of Cushing's disease do not have a history of undetectable 72-hours post-operative serum cortisol levels. Therefore, if 72-hours post-operative cortisol levels are not below 5 µg/dL, further investigations are warranted to confirm cure.

What are the management options of this condition?

The treatment choice for Cushing's disease is transsphenoidal surgery performed by designated Pituitary neurosurgeons. In cases where surgery is not possible or has failed, patients can be treated with medical therapy (ketoconazole), radiation or adrenalectomy.

Potential debates for discussion

- Problems with total hypophysectomy (for the treatment of Cushing's disease) in young patients.
- Role of radiotherapy in Nelson's syndrome.

Case 10C

A 47-year-old man reports headaches, fatigue, and joint pain. His past medical history includes hypertension and carpal tunnel syndrome. He has been diagnosed with acromegaly.

What investigations should be performed for this condition?

The diagnosis of acromegaly should be confirmed. Obtain a detailed history and examine the cardiovascular, respiratory and neurological systems. Collaboration with an endocrinologist is recommended. Further investigations include general and specific investigations.

General tests

- Full blood count, urea and electrolytes, urine dipstick (assess for glucose: diabetes), chest radiography and ECG.

Specific tests

- Pituitary function test (e.g. prolactin, 8 am cortisol, FSH, LH, T4, TSH, IGF-1, fasting glucose).
- Growth hormone (GH): In acromegaly GH >10 ng/mL.
- IGF-1 (somatomedin): In acromegaly IGF-1> 6.8 U/mL.
- Glucose suppression test (oral glucose tolerance test [GTT]): Give 75 mg of glucose to the patient and then measure the serum GH levels every 30 minutes for 2 hours. Positive test for acromegaly >5 mcg/L.
- Visual field assessment.

- Brain MRI scan.
- Further assessment: Colonoscopy (due to increased risk of colonic polyps).

What are the management options of this condition?

Acromegaly should be managed by transsphenoidal surgery. Surgery provides a more rapid reduction in GH levels and decompresses the neural structures. In cases where surgery is not possible or has failed, patients can be treated with medical therapy. Dopamine agonists (bromocriptine, pegvisomant or octreotide) should be used. Radiation is reserved for patients in whom medical treatment has failed and should not be considered as an initial treatment.

Potential debates for discussion

- Role of octreotide as a pre-operative adjunct.
- Criteria for 'cure'.
- Use of fractionated radiotherapy vs. gamma knife radiosurgery for relapses of acromegaly following surgery.

Case 10D

A 29-year-old man presents with new onset of seizures coupled with headaches. He has been diagnosed with arteriovenous malformation (AVM).

What are the management options for this condition?

Management is based on the following:

- Age of the patient.
- Comorbidities.
- Associated aneurysms (on feeding vessels, draining veins or intra-nidal).
- Flow (high or low).
- History of previous haemorrhage.
- Size and compactness of the nidus.
- Patient's wishes.

Treatment options for AVMs are conservative, medical, endovascular and surgical. Surgery is the treatment choice for low-grade AVMs. The Spetzler–Martin classification grades AVMs according to their degree of surgical difficulty and the risk of surgical morbidity and mortality. The Spetzler–Martin AVM grading system allocates points for various features of intracranial AVMs to provide an overall score between 1 and 5. Grade 6 is used to describe inoperable lesions.

Eloquence of adjacent brain

Eloquence of brain: Sensorimotor, language, visual cortex, hypothalamus, thalamus, brain stem, cerebellar nuclei or regions directly adjacent to these structures.

Non-eloquence of brain: Frontal and temporal lobe, cerebellar hemispheres.

Low-grade AVM:	Grade I, II, III
High-grade AVM:	Grade IV, V
Inoperative lesions:	Grade VI

Spetzler–Martin grading system

Size of nidus

Small (<3 cm)	= 1
Medium (3–6 cm)	= 2
Large (> 6 cm)	= 3

Eloquence of adjacent brain

Non-eloquent	= 0
Eloquent	= 1

Venous drainage

Superficial only	= 0
Deep	= 1

Three-tier classification of cerebral AVMs with treatment paradigm (2011).

Class	Spetzler–Martin Grade	Management
A	I and II	Resection
B	III	Multimodality treatment
C	IV and V	No treatment

Potential debates for discussion

- Results for epilepsy control after stereotactic radiosurgery (STRS) for AVMs.
- Influence of combined endovascular embolization on obliteration rates after STRS for AVMs.
- Discussion of the Randomized Trial of Unruptured Brain Arteriovenous Malformation (ARUBA) study and its potential limitations.

References

Spetzler M, Martin N. A proposed grading system for arteriovenous malformations. *J Neurosurg* 1986; 65: 476–483.

Spetzler RF, Ponce FA. A 3-tier classification of cerebral arteriovenous malformations. Clinical article. *J Neurosurg* 2011; *114*(3): 842–849.

Case 10E

A 45-year-old woman presents with unilateral hearing loss and tinnitus. She has been diagnosed with vestibular schwannoma.

What are the management options for this condition?

The treatment options for vestibular schwannomas are conservative, radiation and surgical.

The two most popular management options have the following profiles.

Microsurgery

- >97% chance of complete tumour removal.
- 95% of patients with small tumours retaining House–Brackmann grade I or II facial function.
- 50% retaining useful hearing.

Radiosurgery

- 90% of cases: Vestibular schwannoma will stop growing.
- 98% of cases: No facial nerve palsy.
- 75% will retain useful hearing.

The major determinants of which treatment is adopted are the following:

- Tumour size.
- Age of the patient.
- Comorbidities.
- Hearing preservation.
- State of the hearing in the contralateral ear.
- Patient's wishes.

Potential debates for discussion

- Hearing assessment.
- Management of bilateral vestibular schwannomas in neurofibromatosis type II (NF-2) cases for tumour control and hearing preservation.

Reference

Rutherford SA, King AT. Vestibular schwannoma management: what is the "best" options? *Br J Neurosurg* 2005; *19*(4): 309–316.

Case 10F

A 17-year-old boy presents with a 2-week history of progressive headaches associated with nausea and vomiting. His brain MRI scan demonstrates a homogeneous and hyper-intense mass in the pineal region with associated hydrocephalus.

What are the management options for this condition?

Initial management of patients with pineal region tumours should be directed at treating the underlying hydrocephalus and establishing a diagnosis of the underlying pineal tumour. The treatment of hydrocephalus depends on the patient's clinical state and subsequent definitive treatment plan. Options include close observation while awaiting surgery, ventriculoscopy or EVD, endoscopic third ventriculostomy (ETV), or a VP shunt. A third ventriculostomy has the added advantage of potentially allowing for an open biopsy during the procedure by endoscopic guidance.

Pre-operative evaluation should include the following:

- A high-resolution brain MRI scan with gadolinium.

Spine MRI
- Measurement of serum and CSF markers (by LP, if no contraindication or by ventricular access).
- Cytology examination of CSF.
- Evaluation of pituitary function, if endocrine abnormalities are suspected.
- Visual field examination if suprasellar extension of the tumour is demonstrated on the MRI scan. The ultimate management goal should be to refine adjuvant therapy based on tumour pathology.

Serum and CSF tumour markers as follows.

Alpha-fetoprotein is commonly elevated in the following:

- Yolk sac tumours.
- Embryonal cell carcinoma.
- Immature teratoma.

Beta-human chorionic gonadotropin is commonly elevated in the following:

- Choriocarcinoma.
- Germinoma with syncytiotrophoblasts.
- Embryonal cell carcinomas.

Placental alkaline phosphatase is commonly elevated in the following:

Germinomas.
- May be positive in all germ cell tumours (GCTs).

The management steps depend upon the presence or absence of hydrocephalus and the degree of raised ICP (clinically). Those patients in coma and who have hydrocephalus need an urgent EVD. Those patients who are stable with hydro-cephalus require serum tumour markers, spinal MRI scan and commencement of dexamethasone. Await results of the patient's serum markers and then proceed with a third ventriculostomy and endoscopic biopsy. Also obtain CSF for tumour markers. No need to perform a biopsy if there are positive serum markers or multifocal pineal + suprasellar involvement. In the latter group after ETV, proceed with cycles of chemo-RT with interval radiological assessment. If there is a residual mass, proceed to a surgical resection. In the first group if biopsy confirmed germinoma, the treatment is chemo-RT (modern recommendations add chemotherapy). If other pathologies and absence of spinal or leptomeningeal spread, consider resection. The resection and its extent depend on the histological type, age, comorbidities and configuration of the tumour. The choice of operative approach depends on craniocaudal extent of the lesion and other anatomical constraints for the trajectory and the experience of the surgeon. Those lesions without hydrocephalus obtain serum and CSF via LP for tumour markers and arrange a spinal MRI scan. When considering surveillance, evaluate the patient's clinical presentation, MRI appearances and patient factors. Interval MRI scans are arranged to assess disease progression. Otherwise consider stereotactic or open biopsy and proceed accordingly.

The common surgical approaches include infratentorial supracerebellar, occipital transtentorial and transcallosal interhemispheric. Radiotherapy is indicated for all patients with germinomas, malignant GCTs, malignant or intermediate pineal cell tumours, anaplastic gliomas, or subtotal resection of pineocytoma or ependymomas. Chemotherapy (usually combined with radiotherapy) is used in germinoma, non-germinomatous GCTs, germinoma with syncytiotrophoblastic cells and recurrent or metastatic germinoma or pineal cell tumours.

Potential debates for discussion

- Diagnosis and management of incidental pineal cysts.
- Role of tumour markers in precluding a tissue diagnosis.
- Likely diagnosis (statistically) and management in a patient with a pineal tumour and elevated β-HCG levels.

Case 10G

A 55-year-old woman presents with a sudden onset of a severe headache coupled with vomiting and photophobia. Her head CT scan demonstrates an extensive SAH.

What are the management options of this condition?

The patient is treated with hypervolemia, hypertension and haemodilution. Nimodipine (60 mg PO every 4 hours for 21 days) should be commenced. If there is clinical and radiological evidence of hydrocephalus, an EVD should be inserted. Further investigations include computed tomography angiography (CTA), transcranial Doppler and a formal cerebral angiogram. Treatment is conservative, medical, endovascular or surgical. In patients with a ruptured intracranial aneurysm, the outcome (survival free of disability at 1 year) is better with endovascular coiling compared to clipping.

	Endovascular (%)	Surgery (%)
Dependent or dead at 1 year	23.7	30.6
Relative and absolute risk reductions in dependency or death	22.6	6–9

What is the grading system for SAH?

Hunt and Hess grading

Grade	Clinical condition
0	Unruptured
I	Asymptomatic or minimal headache, nuchal rigidity
II	Moderate to severe headache, nuchal rigidity, no neurological deficit other than cranial nerve palsy
III	Drowsiness, confusion, mild focal deficit
IV	Stupor, moderate to severe hemiparesis, possible early decerebrate rigidity and vegetative disturbances
V	Deep coma, decerebrate rigidity, moribund appearance

World Federation of Neurological Surgeons (WFNS) grading

WFNS grades	GCS score	Motor deficit
I	15	Absent
II	14–13	Absent
III	14–13	Present
IV	12–7	Present or absent
V	6–3	Present or absent

Reference

Molyneux A, Kerr R, Stratton I et al. (International Subarachnoid Aneurysm Trial [ISAT] Collaborative Group). International Subarachnoid Aneurysm Trial (ISAT) of neurosurgical clipping versus endovascular coiling in 2143 patients with ruptured intracranial aneurysms: a randomised trial. *Lancet* 2002; 360: 1267–1274.

Case 10H

A 53-year-old woman presents with a 3-year history of headaches. She is a smoker and has a family history of cerebral aneurysms.

What is the natural history of unruptured aneurysms?

Risk of rupture depends on the following:

- **Size:** The most important predictor for future rupture.
  - <10 mm in diameter: 0.05%/year.
  - >10 mm in diameter: 1%/year.

A follow-up by the International Study of Unruptured Intracranial Aneurysms Investigators stated the 5-year cumulative rupture rate for patients with unruptured aneurysms.

Size of unruptured aneurysm	<7	7–12	13–24	>24
Anterior circulation	0	2.6	14.5	40%
Posterior circulation	2.5	14.5	18.4	50%

- **Site**: Posterior communicating artery (PCoA), vertebrobasilar and basilar termination unruptured aneurysms are more likely to rupture.
- **Morphology**: Irregular and multi-lobular aneurysms are more likely to rupture.
- The PHASES score is an aid for the prediction of the risk of rupture for asymptomatic intracranial aneurysms.
- PHASES score
  P – Population (e.g. Japanese or Finnish)
  H – Hypertension
  A – Age > 70 years
  S – Size of aneurysm
  E – Earlier SAH from another aneurysm
  S – Site: Anatomical location of aneurysm

What are the principles of screening? In the general population, is there a screening test for cerebral aneurysms?
Principles of screening are a test performed on asymptomatic individuals that allows for early detection, therapeutic intervention and decreased mortality from the disease.

Wilson's criteria (World Health Organization guidelines)

- The condition should be an important health problem.
- The natural history of the condition should be understood.
- There should be a recognizable latent or early symptomatic stage.
- There should be a test that is easy to perform and interpret, acceptable, accurate, reliable, sensitive and specific.
- There should be an accepted treatment recognized for the disease.
- Treatment should be more effective if started early.
- There should be a policy on who should be treated.
- Diagnosis and treatment should be cost-effective.
- Case finding should be a continuous process.

Screening of cerebral aneurysms is not well established.

- The natural history is not known. We do not know how rapidly an aneurysm forms. It may be days, weeks or months. Therefore, even after a negative cerebral angiogram, there is no evidence that an aneurysm will not form.
- Screening technology is not sensitive enough to detect small aneurysms.
- Small aneurysms have a small rupture risk.
- Aneurysm treatment is not without risk.
- Incidental detected aneurysms have repercussions for applications for mortgages and life insurance policies.

Screening in patients with familial intracranial aneurysms is controversial. There is evidence that patients with two or more first-degree relatives who have had aneurysmal bleeds are more likely to have cerebral aneurysms than the baseline population and are generally advised to be screened. Magnetic resonance angiography (MRA) scan is the investigation of choice because it is less invasive and more cost effective compared to cerebral angiography.

Potential debates for discussion

Frequency of serial imaging in unruptured intracranial aneurysms managed conservatively.

References

Wiebers D, Whisnant J, Forbes G et al. (International Study of Unruptured Intracranial Aneurysms Investigators). Unruptured intracranial aneurysms – risk of rupture and risks of surgical intervention. *N Engl J Med* 1998; *339(24)*: 1725–1733.

Wiebers DO, Whisnant JP, Houston J et al. (International Study of Unruptured Intracranial Aneurysms Investigators.) Unruptured intracranial aneurysms: natural history, clinical outcome, and risks of surgical and endovascular treatment. *Lancet* 2003; *362*: 103–110.

6 | Key Illustrative Cases

The following are common cases and practical advice on how to answer the 'hot topics'. We provide a strategy on how to approach each case and highlight the key areas to cover in the examination.

Neurovascular cases

Sylvian ICH – Ruptured MCA aneurysm

Safety – Predict variations: Specific precautions

If there are no further details about the given case, then begin by mentioning the key factors that determine the management of a ruptured aneurysm. The key factors include the patient's GCS, their rate of deterioration, the patient's age, size of haematoma and evidence of mass effect. In patients with low GCS, who rapidly deteriorated, and harbour a large intracerebral haematoma (ICH), then the priority is to treat the increased intracranial pressure (ICP) by medical optimization (e.g. administration of mannitol) followed by craniotomy to evacuate the haematoma and clip the underlying aneurysm. Your answer should be tailored to the specific case and demonstrate your safe approach, avoidance of complications, surgical anatomical knowledge and experience. Pre-operative planning should include an understanding of the haematoma (location) and the aneurysm (size and projection of the fundus). Planning the head position on the operation table with the size of the craniotomy flap will allow for adequate ICH decompression and the ability to obtain safe proximal control. When evacuating the ICH, be safe and try and prevent aneurysm rerupture. Depending on the anatomical location of the clot, evacuation can be achieved by splitting the distal sylvian fissure away from the expected aneurysm to allow for a trans-sylvian evacuation. In cases of large dominant hemisphere temporal clots, a trans-superior temporal gyrus approach with an anterior corticotomy may be more appropriate. In either case, the initial evacuation should be partial so as not to disturb the tamponade effect of the clot on the underlying aneurysm but large enough to allow for brain relaxation and access to the basal cisterns for proximal control. Once the aneurysm is clipped, the residual ICH can be evacuated.

If the aneurysm size and configuration are favourable, demonstrate your anatomical knowledge and safety by describing how you would clip the aneurysm. This could include proximal control, dissection of M1, use of temporary clips (preferably distal to the lenticulostriate branch), identification of all M2 branches (look carefully for extra branches – trifurcation rather than bifurcation), circumferential fundus dissection

DOI: 10.1201/9781003254379-6

and assurance that the clip does not occlude or kink any associated branches. The use of intraoperative indocyanine green (ICG) is helpful in these situations.

If you choose to evacuate the ICH and then proceed to endovascular coiling, mention the key safety steps to prevent intraoperative rupture. Following endovascular coiling, be prepared to advise on the potential benefits and complications of periprocedural heparin and antiplatelet agents.

If faced with a ruptured giant aneurysm, a safe option is to perform a decompressive craniectomy. Once the patient has been stabilized, an experienced vascular neurosurgeon can take over the patient's care. If you report preservation of the superficial temporal artery while performing the craniotomy, then proceeding to partial ICH evacuation to allow for brain relaxation, gaining proximal control, dissecting the aneurysm neck, preserving all M2 branches and proceeding to bypass is not the ideal answer. Giant aneurysms should be referred to an experienced vascular surgeon in a multidisciplinary setting, and not addressed by a junior neurosurgeon.

In stable patients, a further option is to select endovascular coiling of the aneurysm followed by evacuation of the ICH, if required. Demonstrate awareness regarding the use of anticoagulants during the procedure and their reversal prior to craniotomy.

Case 1: A 28-year-old pregnant woman presents with WFNS grade I subarachnoid haemorrhage (SAH) from a ruptured 7-mm internal carotid bifurcation aneurysm

Awareness of variations – Safety

The key to this case is to focus on the management of the SAH and consider the influence of the pregnancy on the recommended treatments.

The management options (e.g. conservative, medical, endovascular and surgical) depend on patient selection and the underlying aneurysm. During the first trimester, there is a potentially high risk of teratogenic effects of medication and anaesthesia on the fetus. At term, consideration for an elective caesarean section followed by surgery may be the best treatment. There is no standard answer because each patient is different. If endovascular treatment is chosen, be specific in mentioning shielding the fetus from radiation, positioning the patient (tilting the abdomen to the left side to decrease the compression of the inferior vena cava) and involving the obstetricians.

Case 2: A 65-year-old man presents with perimesencephalic SAH. The computed tomography angiography (CTA) scan does not demonstrate a vascular abnormality

Awareness of controversy – Principles of management

The definition of what constitutes perimesencephalic SAH is debatable. Digital subtraction angiography (DSA) remains the gold standard in diagnosing aneurysms.

Be prepared for debate. Acknowledge the possible diagnostic challenges. Most surgeons would recommend DSA. In the context of perimesencephalic SAH with a negative initial DSA, this would not require further investigations. In practice, management can be complex. For example, if the patient has evidence of interhemispheric extension (which by definition is minor and still classifies the bleed as a perimesencephalic type), the decision whether or not to repeat an angiography to exclude anterior communicating aneurysm (ACoA) is not clear.

Case 3: Counselling a 32-year-old teacher who is diagnosed with an incidental 14-mm anterior communicating aneurysm

Comprehensive – Only relevant figures: Very specific treatment risks

The counselling includes three discussions: (1) the natural history of the vascular lesion; (2) treatment options with the associated benefits and complications and (3) the psychological impact on the patient. There are two parts to the consultation: information giving (explaining the diagnosis) and information gathering (exploring the patient's views and specific worries).

When discussing the natural history of this condition, mention the risk of rupture based on evidence provided by the International Study of Unruptured Intracranial Aneurysm (ISUIA) study (in reference to the size of an anterior circulation aneurysm [see table]), PHASES score and a multidisciplinary consensus on the unruptured aneurysm treatment score.

Size of aneurysm	Anterior circulation	Posterior circulation
	% of rupture rates	% of rupture rates
< 7 mm	0	2.5
7–12 mm	2.6	14.5
13–24 mm	14.5	18.4
≥25 mm	40	50

Mention the limitations of the study and that the life-long risks still need to be calculated. Added factors that increase the risk of rupture in addition to size are irregular shape/daughter lobule, smoking, uncontrolled hypertension, family history, possible association with polycystic kidney disease, previous SAH from unrelated aneurysm and progressive increase in size. In addition, shear stress studies and vascular wall imaging are currently research tools trying to add additional information to estimate further risk factors. The risk is adjusted to the age of the patient. This patient is 32 years old with a possible increased risk due to the location of the aneurysm (ACoA aneurysms) and gender (female).

Best to be specific in explaining the potential risks of treatment that apply directly to the ACoA aneurysm. Discuss the positive morphological factors in obtaining long-term obliteration rates.

PHASES score is an aid for the predication of the risk of rupture for asymptomatic intracranial aneurysms:

P – Population – (e.g. Japanese or Finnish).
H – Hypertension.

A – Age > 70 years.
S – Size of the aneurysm.
E – Earlier SAH from another aneurysm.
S – Site: Anatomical location of aneurysm.

Case 4: A 43-year-old man has recovered well following an SAH. He underwent endovascular coiling of a posterior communicating artery (PCoA) aneurysm with a fetal PCoA. At 6 months, his MRI/MRA scans demonstrated a recurrence and partial filling of the aneurysm neck

Awareness of controversy – Specific precautions

Demonstrate knowledge regarding the overall incidence of recurrence and factors that increase these rates. In the long-term, re-canalization and recurrence occur overall in about 20–30% (recurrences and progression of residual neck filling). Those with large residuals, recurrences, progression and those presenting with bleeding from the residual aneurysm require further treatment; this occurs in about 10–15% of cases. The majority of minor, stable residuals or recurrences require only followed-up surveillance, especially in younger patients. Factors that increase recurrence rates include smoking, the end result after initial coiling, neck configuration, packing density of the coils, presence of intra-aneurysmal thrombus, length of follow-up with special consideration for age and interval for the recurrence and possibly certain locations.

Safety is a major component of this clinical examination. Before embarking on any treatment options, assess the natural history of the condition. Discuss the different patterns of recurrence, filling of the fundus and, more importantly, the known rebleeding risk from the recurrent or residual neck. If you decide to quote figures from the literature, be aware that there are wide variations in different series.

If re-coiling of the aneurysm is the best option, then demonstrate the possible complications, including the need for stent-assisted recoiling and the importance of not occluding the dominant PCoA. The role of surgical clipping should also be mentioned. This may be suitable in cases where there is evidence of coil impaction. Surgery would allow for the application of the aneurysmal clip without retrieval of the coils whilst preserving the PCoA. Clipping, although technically challenging, would provide a better long-term outcome.

Case 5: A 16-year-old boy presents with controlled seizures and has been diagnosed with a deep insular 2-cm AVM

Safety – Defend treatment option: Specific results

The key to the questions is that the patient is young with a deep-seated vascular lesion. The life-long risk of bleeding from this AVM will need a discussion. The primary aim of treatment is to curtail the risk of bleeding rather than to obtain seizure control. A Randomized Trial of Unruptured Brain Arteriovenous Malformation (ARUBA) interim analysis demonstrated that medical management is superior to intervention in patients with unruptured AVMs. However, the result is applied mostly to the endovascular intervention arm of treatment. *Be safe*: Surgery for deep-seated AVMs has serious potential complications. Stereotactic radiosurgery can be considered in small AVMs.

Case 6: An 18-year-old woman, who underwent childhood cranial radiation for leukaemia, presents with sudden onset of upper limb clumsiness, a sensory deficit in the lower face and diplopia. Her head MRI scan demonstrates a pontine cavernoma with minor haemorrhage

Knowledge – Management options: Safety

Consider the young age of this patient in the context of the natural history of brainstem cavernomas. Because the patient has undergone previous whole brain radiation, stereotactic radiation may not be an ideal recommendation.

Focus on safety. Delayed surgery may be advantageous as a further episode of haemorrhage will create a gliotic plane allowing for an improved surgical corridor. Mention the specific factors, including location within the pons and the characteristics of the haemorrhage (e.g. whether the bleed presents to the cortical surface or is surrounded by functional neural tissue). Without prompting by the examiner, state that any associated developmental venous anomaly (DVA) should remain untouched.

Demonstrate your neuroanatomical knowledge by indicating the safe surgical approaches and illustrate the position of the various nuclei and tracts on the floor of the fourth ventricle, as shown in Figure 6.1.

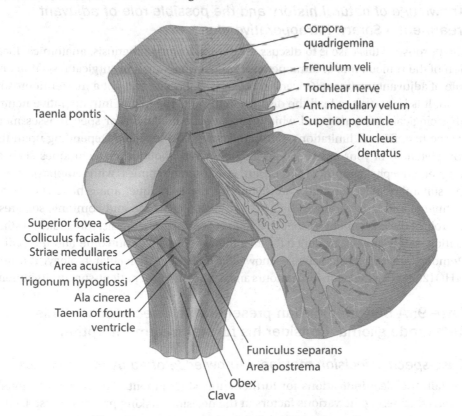

Figure 6.1 Anatomy of the fourth ventricle (Case 6).

Tumour cases

Case 7: A 52-year-old man presents with a typical history of migraines. His head MRI scan demonstrates a 12-mm colloid cyst with no associated hydrocephalus

Knowledge – Specific advice to the patient: Specific approach

Demonstrate your knowledge regarding the overall management of incidental colloid cysts. This should include the accepted recommendation for treatment if the colloid cyst is symptomatic, >10 mm in size and located high in the septum pellucidum or in the roof of the third ventricle. Sudden death due to a colloid cyst is rare, but it is important in counselling the patient. Discuss the significance of the presence or absence of hydrocephalus in selecting a surgical approach. Safety is the major key issue; do not underestimate the morbidity (including memory impairment) and mortality following transcallosal surgery.

In this case, take into consideration the history of migraines, which would be problematic if a conservative approach is adopted. If the patient is treated conservatively, advise the patient to seek urgent medical attention if symptoms progress.

Case 8: A 43-year-old woman is diagnosed with a left-sided low-grade glioma in the opercular part of the inferior frontal gyrus

Knowledge of natural history and the possible role of adjuvant treatment – Safety: Intraoperative plan

The purpose of this case is to discuss the natural history, prognosis, anatomical location of the tumour, role of intraoperative monitoring, extent of surgical resection and role of adjuvant treatment. Cover the basics well. Be safe and not a master neurosurgeon. It is important to lead the discussion towards the role of intraoperative neurophysiological monitoring and white matter tract stimulation for speech assessment vs. the benefits and limitations of intraoperative MRI imaging. Depending upon the completeness of your answers, you may be asked about other techniques such as magnetoencephalography (MEG) with awake craniotomies with emphasis upon the suitability, selection and counselling for the technique, anaesthetic sequence/technique and intraoperative challenges (e.g. pain, agitation and vomiting, seizures), the role of the assessment by speech therapist/neuropsychologists, thresholds of stimulation, safety and the evidence for its influence on patient outcome and morbidity. Demonstrate your basic science knowledge regarding molecular biology, the new WHO (2021) Classification for Tumours and the potential for patient-specific treatment.

Case 9: A 56-year-old man presents with a recurrence in his high-grade glioma. Consider his further treatment options

Case-specific decision-making – Knowledge of adjuvant therapies

Explain the clear indications for further surgical treatment. Explain your rationale when considering the various factors in the decision-making process. These factors include age, performance status, interval to recurrence, response to previous treatment, patient's expectations, availability of further adjuvant treatment options, accessibility for further resection, safety of further surgery and prediction of resectability. The first step is to confirm that the lesion is recurrent tumour rather than radionecrosis. Imaging can be helpful in these diagnostic dilemmas, which include the various diagnostic modalities with their sensitivities, specificities and limitations (e.g. positron emission tomography [PET], perfusion MRI scans) into your explanation. For a patient undergoing further surgery, the use of Gliadel wafers (prolifeprosan 20 with carmustine implant) may be considered. Be aware of the benefits, side effects, limitations and contraindications to their use. Discuss the role of glioma biomarkers in classifying and grading gliomas. The overall survival or progression-free survival is longer in patients with O(6)-methylguanine-DNA methyltransferase (MGMT) promoter methylation and *IDH-1* mutations. This is an opportunity to demonstrate current, evidence-based literature to support management options.

Epilepsy case

Case 10: A 27-year-old university lecturer presents with three to four uncontrolled seizures per month. His underlying diagnosis is presumed to be hippocampal sclerosis. Perform an adequate pre-operative assessment

Individual considerations – Relevant assessment for surgery: Understanding investigations

Before answering the question, consider the relevant facts that have been provided. It is best to avoid the obvious pitfall by stating that you will establish the patient's seizure frequency and recommend management according to the patient's age and occupation. These are facts that have already been provided. Do not waste valuable time repeating established facts.

Because the question mentions a pre-operative assessment, it is fair to say that you would reconfirm the indications for surgery by taking a detailed history, performing a neurological examination and reviewing all investigations. Nevertheless, as a neurosurgeon mention the importance of establishing that the seizures are 'true' rather than 'pseudo' seizures understand the semiology of the seizures, ensure that the patient was compliant in taking anticonvulsants, ensure that sufficient time was afforded for medical optimization and determine the patient's overall quality of life. The question indicates that the assessment has been performed, but it is important to confirm the diagnosis, localize the target and report on the safety of surgery. The initial workup includes blood tests, a brain MRI scan and electroencephalography (EEG) with video telemetry. Discussion may also include different MRI sequences and hippocampal volume assessment. If there is doubt regarding the localization of the lesion, discuss the role, principles and limitations of ictal and interictal PET, single-photon emission computed tomography (SPECT) and subdural and depth electrodes. In addition, demonstrate an understanding of functional magnetic resonance imaging (fMRI) and the Wada test. The patient's speech, memory and neuropsychological state will also need to be assessed.

In summary, these steps ensure the indications for surgery, localizing the appropriate target and maintaining safety by minimizing potential morbidity (including memory dysfunction) and mortality.

Spine case

Case 11: A 56-year-old woman presents with bilateral leg pain and low back pain. Her lumbar MRI scan demonstrates a L4/L5 spondylolisthesis

Dealing with grey areas – Classification: Operative options – Outcomes

Spine surgery is one of the least clear-cut areas of neurosurgery. There is great variation in practice. In cases, where there can be a lack of consensus, discuss the available different treatments options whilst explaining their potential advantages and disadvantages. Involve the spinal multidisciplinary team is reasonable. Regarding the patient's history and examination, there are some key features to identify. Clearly, the presence of significant radicular symptoms and signs would support intervention. As a lumbar decompression may result in spinal instability, lumbar fusion (instrumented fixation +/– interbody cage) is now accepted practice. When considering a fusion, assess patient's factors (e.g. smoking, steroids, osteoporotic fractures, nonsteroidal anti-inflammatory medication, rheumatoid arthritis, Parkinson's disease, diabetes mellitus, malnutrition, immunosuppression, etc.).

Recommended imaging is a lumbar MRI scan, lumbar CT scan and lumbar radiographs (standing or flexion/extension studies). In fact, whole spine radiographs can assess the patient's over spinal parameters (sagittal balance, pelvic incidence [PI]).

- Sagittal balance is determined by the C7 plump line which is a vertical line drawn from the centre of the C7 vertebral body running parallel to the edge of the radiograph. The normal C7 plumb line passes within millimetres of the posterior-superior corner of S1. Positive sagittal balance occurs when the C7 plumb line falls anterior to the posterior-superior corner of the S1 endplate. Negative sagittal balance occurs when the C7 plumb line falls posterior to this point (Figure 6.2).
- **PI**: Pelvic tilt (PT) + sacral slope (SS). These angles are parameters used to describe the shape and orientation of the pelvis conditioning spinal sagittal balance.
  - **PT**: A vertical line through the femoral head and line from the mid-sacral plateau and femoral head
  - **SS**: An angle between a horizontal line and the orientation of the sacral plateau (Figure 6.3)

When reporting the imaging, mention the presence or absence of a pars defect and the Meyerding classification (Figures 6.4 and 6.5).

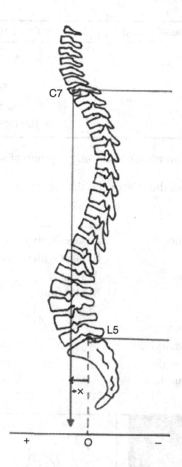

Figure 6.2 Sagittal balance.

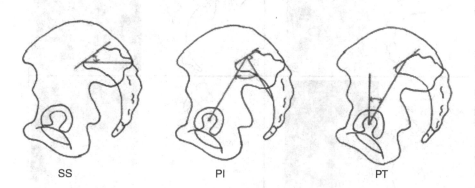

Figure 6.3 Sacral slope, pelvic incidence, pelvic tilt (PI = PT + SS).

Meyerding classification	Percentage of slip
Grade I	0–25
Grade II	25–50
Grade III	50–75
Grade IV	75–100
Grade V	> 100 (spondyloptosis)

Figure 6.4 The Meyerding classification system of spondylolisthesis.

One should also be aware of the Wiltse classification:

Type		
I	Dysplastic	A: facet with axial orientation
		B: facet with sagittal orientation
II	Isthmic	A: lysis
		B: elongation
		C: fracture
III	Degenerative	
IV	Post-traumatic	
V	Pathologic	
VI	Postsurgical	

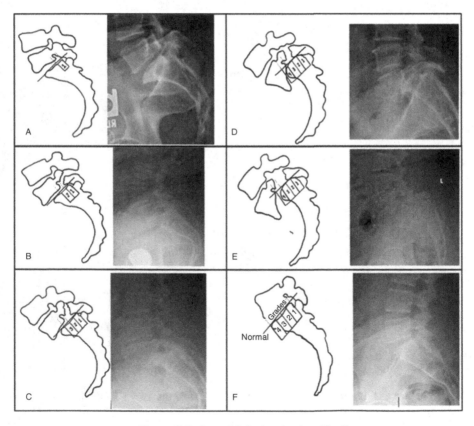

Figure 6.5 Spondylolisthesis classification.

Examiners may go on to discuss factors that increase the risk of developing spondylolisthesis (e.g. high PI, sagittally oriented facets, etc.).

Regarding management, it is relevant publications to support management choices. In the case of lumbar spondylolisthesis, The SPORT study demonstrated the superiority of surgery at 2 and 4 years post-operatively. The Swedish Spinal Stenosis Study found that with lumbar canal stenosis, with or without degenerative spondylolisthesis, there was no difference in clinical outcome with fusion compared with decompression alone. There are also studies showing no difference in outcome with physiotherapy alone vs. surgery.

When considering lumbar fusions, there are many techniques to choose from Buck's screws, ALIF, TLIF, XLIF, OLIF and posterolateral screws. Examiners are not expecting detailed knowledge about a novel technique. Best to explain posterior instrumented fusion with pedicle screws should be sufficient – e.g. entry points, trajectories and insertion techniques (e.g. free-hand, X-ray, O-arm or robotic guided).

The complexities of sagittal balance are probably beyond the remit of neurosurgery exit exams, but one should at least express awareness that attention to maintaining sagittal balance is important even in a single-level fixation. It is also important to monitor your outcomes with pre- and post-operative questionnaires: Visual Analogue Scores (VASs) and Oswestry Disability Index (ODI) scores with a submission to a National Registry such as the British Spine Registry.

Paediatric case

Case 12: The neonatal unit refers a baby with spina bifida

Dealing with an unfamiliar situation – Controversies: Emerging techniques

There are quite specific approaches that would be expected in dealing with paediatric cases that may not be familiar to one's general practice. Establishing the patient's pre- and peri-natal history:

- Pre-natal or ante-natal diagnosis?
- Type of delivery
- Gestational age
- APGAR score
- Other suspected defects (VACTERL)
- Family history of spina bifida
- Pregnancy history
- Spina bifida occulta or aperta?

There might be discussions on pre-natal investigation. Knowledge of usual schedule for maternal ultrasound is useful. When would sampling of amniotic fluid be considered? What supplements are advised in pregnancy?

One should have a schema for examining the baby:

- Examination of each neural arch (from the cervical to the sacral region)
- Is the defect covered by skin?
- Is there evidence of CSF leak?
- Are there associated syndromic features?
- Orthopaedic assessment: Bilateral talipes, bilateral hip dislocation
- Neuro-examination
  - GCS
  - Anterior fontanelle
  - Check cranial sutures
  - OFC and document to HC chart (corrected by age)
  - Look for enlarged scalp veins
  - Primitive reflexes
  - Muscle tone (ASWORTH modified scale)
  - Bladder function: Are the diapers/nappies constantly wet?
  - Tolerating feed

Immediate management would include nursing the baby prone and covering the defect with a sterile saline-soaked dressing. Attention to avoid hypothermia. These babies are liable to latex allergy, and a latex free environment should be maintained. Antibiotics are indicated. Intermittent catheterization should be considered in cases with a neuropathic bladder.

Investigations would include the following:

- Whole neuro-axis MRI scan (Establish and assess for the level of defect, Arnold Chiari II malformation and hydrocephalus).
- Cranial ultrasound.
- Urodynamic studies.
- Renal ultrasound.

Consider shunting if hydrocephalus is present. Should this be performed at the same time as myelomeningocele repair? Is there evidence? There may be discussions around ETV in infancy and the ETV success score. Although in-depth familiarity with in utero closure would not be expected, the longer-term management under a multi-disciplinary team may also be included.

Guide to prepare controversial topics

It is important to emphasize that the purpose of the Viva component of the exam is to test the application of your knowledge for tailored decision-making for the specific case or situation and execution of the management in a safe and efficient manner. The factual knowledge is assessed through the written or MCQ component of the examination. Bearing in mind the Dreyfus model[1] of adult skill acquisition, the level of the exam is likely to assess your approach to decision-making and selection of management based on your level of experience, and you should, in turn, reflect the degree of application a practice based upon evidence-base medicine and safe management.

Hence, it is most likely that you will be presented with controversial topics for which you are required to select an appropriate treatment after demonstrating the case for and the case against each choice. For this, you need a strategy:

- Be aware of the case for and the case against each option.
- The factors and variables you need to consider for making this decision.
- Justify the application of the selected option specifically to the given situation or case.

The following is a list of interesting and datable topics. This is to alert you to prepare yourself while reading and you may return back to this list as you advance with your preparation. This is by no means a comprehensive list. For this list below, find the relevant key publications that support either side of the case. Prepare a list of the variables that you would consider in your decision-making.

- The case for and against the use of prophylactic anticonvulsant in different types of conditions (e.g. trauma, infection and tumour surgery).
- The use of mannitol vs. hypertonic saline in the control of elevated ICP.
- The need, duration and frequency of routine follow-up imaging for incidental lesions (e.g. small colloid cysts, incidental cavernomas and unruptured aneurysms).
- Awake craniotomy vs. the use of intraoperative MRI scans for resection of low-grade gliomas and other intrinsic lesions involving eloquent areas.
- Application or omission of whole brain radiation with stereotactic radiosurgery (SRS), surgical resection or focused radiotherapy (RT) for multiple brain metastases.
- The case for and against and selection for pre-operative embolization in meningioma surgery.
- Application of upfront RT after different degrees of resection of WHO grade 2 meningiomas.
- Endoscopic endonasal vs. transcranial approaches for tuberculum sellae/planum sphenoidale meningiomas.
- Management of craniopharyngiomas: Extent of resection and approaches.
- Open vs. endoscopic resection of colloid cysts.
- Supracerebellar infratentorial vs. occipital trans-tentorial approaches to pineal lesions.
- Retrosigmoid vs. translabrynthine approach for vestibular schwannomas.
- Conservative vs. SRS vs. surgery for small vestibular schwannomas with intact hearing.
- Endoscopic resection of ethesioneuroblastomas.
- Hypothermia in the management of severe TBI.
- Drain vs. no drain after drainage of chronic subdural haematomas (CSDH).
- Routine post-operative imaging following drainage of CSDH.
- Bone flap removal after craniotomy and evacuation of traumatic acute subdural hematoma (ASDH).
- ACDF with or without additional anterior cervical plating.
- Timing of decompression for spinal cord injury.
- Micro- vs. minimally invasive spine surgery (MISS) vs. endoscopic lumbar discectomy.

- Upfront vs. at recurrence fixation for synovial cysts.
- Management of asymptomatic syrinx and Chiari malformation.
- Microsurgical clipping vs. coiling of intracranial aneurysms.
- Treatment of unruptured AVMs.
- The role of STRS in the management of cavernomas
- Decompressive craniotomy for stroke in the elderly.
- Carotid endarterectomy (CEA) vs. stenting for extracranial carotid disease.
- Deep brain stimulation: Pallidum vs. STN as surgical targets in movement disorders.
- Preservation of vein of Dandy in microvascular decompression.

7 Landmark Publications

In Neurosurgery, a number of publications have changed out practice and decision-making in complex clinical scenarios. Some landmark publications can be asked directly or indirectly in the oral or clinical examinations or can be encountered in MCQ/EMQ exams. Key points of important publications are discussed in the section along with some critiques, where applicable. A list of other important publications are found at the end of this chapter.

Vascular neurosurgery

Timing of aneurysm surgery

The International Cooperative Study on the Timing of Aneurysm Surgery was the first large-scale study to look at this issue. A total of 3521 patients were recruited out of 8879 patients with subarachnoid haemorrhage (SAH). In addition to looking at the timing aspect of surgery, many other factors that influence outcome were addressed.

Kassell *et al.* published "The International Cooperative Study on the Timing of Aneurysm Surgery" in Part 1 – Overall management results and in Part 2 – Surgical results in the *Journal of Neurosurgery* in 1990. Between December 1980 and July 1983, patients having ≤3 days since first SAH from a saccular aneurysm (CT/lumbar puncture (LP) confirmation of bleed, angio/surgical confirmation of aneurysm) were included. Patients with delayed admission >3 days since bleed; multiple bleeds; no confirmation of aneurysm on angio or surgery were excluded.

The main conclusions from this study are that 75% of those admitted within 3 days are in good condition, with a 58% good recovery at 6 months and 25% death rate. Vasospasm and re-bleeding were the major causes of death or disability, aside from the initial effects of the bleed. Few prognostic factors were identified which included admission GCS (patients who were alert pre-operatively had a more favourable overall prognosis if their operation occurred between days 0 and 3 or after day 10) and age (90% good result in the 18–29 years age group vs. 56% in the 60–69 year age group).

Study references

Kassell NF, Torner JC, Haley EC Jr, Jane JA, Adams HP, Kongable GL. The International Cooperative Study on the Timing of Aneurysm Surgery. Part 1: overall management results. *J Neurosurg* 1990; 73: 18–36.

Kassell NF, Torner JC, Jane JA, Haley EC Jr, Adams HP. The International Cooperative Study on the Timing of Aneurysm Surgery. Part 2: surgical results. *J Neurosurg* 1990; 73: 37–47.

DOI: 10.1201/9781003254379-7

Endovascular coiling vs. aneurysm clipping in ruptured aneurysms

The International Subarachnoid Aneurysm Trial (ISAT) is the most comprehensive study comparing endovascular to surgical treatment in ruptured aneurysms, having the greatest impact on treatment of ruptured aneurysms until now.

Molyneux *et al.* for the ISAT Collaborative Group Molyneux *et al.* published "International Subarachnoid Aneurysm Trial (ISAT) of neurosurgical clipping vs. endovascular coiling in 2143 patients with ruptured intracranial aneurysms: a randomised trial" in *Lancet* in 2002.

The patients who had

- CT or LP proven SAH within 28 days;
- Computed tomography angiogram (CTA) or digital subtraction angiography (DSA) proven aneurysm;
- Good enough clinical state to justify treatment;
- Aneurysms judged to be suitable for either technique agreed by both surgeon and neuroradiologist with equipoise regarding which method would be best and consent was included.

The patients who had

- >28 days since SAH;
- Clinical condition considered unsuitable for either or both treatments;
- Lack of consent; and
- Participation in another SAH trial were excluded.

Results of patients who underwent endovascular coiling, 23.7% were dependent or dead at 1 year compared to 30.6% who had their aneurysm surgically clipped ($p < 0.002$). This led to a relative/absolute risk reduction (ARR) of dependency by 22.6% or death by 6.9% at 1 year. Re-bleeding risk at 1 year was 2 per 1276 patient-years in the endovascular group vs. 0 per 1081 patient-years in the surgical group. The difference was not statistically significant.

The conclusion of this study is the outcome, in terms of survival-free disability, is significantly better with endovascular treatment than with surgical clipping of a ruptured aneurysm.

Critique

One of the major criticisms of ISAT is that in this trial the work of good interventional neuroradiologists was compared to 'average' neurosurgeons rather than those who 'concentrate' on neurovascular surgery. In other words, there is an inherent bias in the recruiting centres as being those that have a strong interventional radiology interest. The ISAT group stated that the trial is a 'pragmatic' trial, i.e., it tries to determine the best outcome in a real-life situation for a patient who is supposed to be transferred to their regional unit for diagnosis and treatment. This trial determines the best option for an 'average patient' and does not study the outcome of 'the best possible surgery versus the best possible endovascular treatment. A second criticism is that the trial is biased towards small anterior circulation aneurysms (97.5%). To be fair, the ISAT investigators have never claimed that the trial indicates that all ruptured aneurysms should be coiled in preference to clipping.

Study reference

Molyneux A, Kerr R, Stratton I, Sandercock P, Clarke M, Shrimpton J, Holman R, for the International Subarachnoid Aneurysm Trial (ISAT) Collaborative Group. International Subarachnoid Aneurysm Trial (ISAT) of neurosurgical clipping vs. endovascular coiling in 2143 patients with ruptured intracranial aneurysms: a randomised trial. *Lancet* 2002; *360*: 1267–1274.

Barrow Ruptured Aneurysm Trial (BRAT)

This is a prospective, randomized trial being conducted in Barrow institute which is famous for vascular neurosurgery. In this trial, clipping was compared to coil embolization. Patients were randomized to treatment on presentation with any non-traumatic SAH. Spetzler *et al.* report the 6-year results of this ongoing with the final goal of a 10-year follow-up, comparing the safety and efficacy of clipping and coiling of aneurysmal SAH.

In contrast to ISAT, Spetzler *et al.* observed over a 6-year period that there appeared to be only a marginal difference in outcome between clipping and coiling for treating anterior circulation aneurysms. But, in the posterior circulation aneurysms, coil embolization was found to have a sustained benefit over surgical clipping. Consistent with the current literature, aneurysm obliteration rates in BRAT were lower for coiling than for clipping. However, no recurrent haemorrhages were known to have occurred in either treatment group 6 years after discharge despite the fact that rehaemorrhage rates were higher after coiling. There is no difference in shunt dependency after SAH among patients treated by endovascular or microsurgical means.

Study reference

Spetzler RF, McDougall CG, Zabramski JM, Albuquerque FC, Hills NK, Russin JJ, Partovi S, Nakaji P, Wallace RC. The Barrow Ruptured Aneurysm trial: 6-year results. *J Neurosurg.* 2015 Sep; *123(3)*:609–17. DOI: 10.3171/2014.9.JNS141749. Epub 2015 Jun 26. PMID: 26115467.

Long-term natural history of unruptured aneurysms (ISUIA trial)

The International Study of Unruptured Intracranial Aneurysms Investigators (ISUIA) was the first large-scale, prospective study looking at the natural history of unruptured aneurysms as well as the risks of treatment of unruptured aneurysms. Factors related to prognosis are elucidated.

For the International Study of Unruptured Intracranial Aneurysms Investigators Wiebers *et al.* published the trial result of "Unruptured intracranial aneurysms: natural history, clinical outcome, and risks of surgical and endovascular treatment" in *Lancet* in 2003.

Patients having one or more unruptured intracranial saccular aneurysms (regardless of symptoms other than rupture, e.g., cranial nerve palsy) and Rankin 1 or 2 (self-caring) after previous rupture (patients may not have had previous rupture) were included.

Patients having fusiform, mycotic or traumatic aneurysms; aneurysm <2 mm; SAH from single ruptured aneurysm or unknown source; unruptured aneurysm that was manipulated prior to study; previous intracranial haemorrhage of unknown cause or untreated structural abnormality; malignant brain tumour and bedridden or unable to communicate when aneurysm identified were excluded.

Results were found as 5-year cumulative rupture rate (5YRR)

1. In aneurysms <7 mm, without any other aneurysms with previous rupture
   - In case of cavernous carotid artery aneurysms and AComm or anterior cerebral artery (ACA) aneurysms, risk is nil.
   - In case of vertebrobasilar, posterior cerebral artery (PCA) or P.comm aneurysms, risk is 2.5%.
2. In aneurysms of 7–12 mm
   - In case of cavernous carotid artery aneurysms, risk is nil.
   - In case of A. Comm or ACA aneurysms, risk is 2.6%.
   - In case of vertebrobasilar, PCA or P.comm aneurysms, risk is 14.5%.
3. In aneurysms of 13–24 mm
   - In case of cavernous carotid artery aneurysms, risk is 3%.
   - In case of A. Comm or ACA aneurysms, risk is 15.5%.
   - In case of vertebrobasilar, PCA or P.comm aneurysms, risk is 18.4%.
4. In aneurysms larger than 24 mm
   - In case of cavernous carotid artery aneurysms, risk is 6.4%.
   - In case of A. Comm or ACA aneurysms, risk is 40%.
   - In case of vertebrobasilar, PCA or P.comm aneurysms, risk is 50%.

ISUIA was criticized for its selection bias. Nevertheless, it has had a profound impact on the decision to treat unruptured aneurysms and proved itself as an important evidence for both the neurosurgeons and the interventionists.

Study reference

Wiebers DO, Whisnant JP, Huston J 3rd, Meissner I, Brown RD Jr, Piepgras DG, Forbes GS, Thielen K, Nichols D, O'Fallon WM, Peacock J, Jaeger L, Kassell NF, Kongable-Beckman GL, Torner JC, for the International Study of Unruptured Intracranial Aneurysms Investigators. Unruptured intracranial aneurysms: natural history, clinical outcome, and risks of surgical and endovascular treatment. *Lancet* 2003; 362: 103–110.

Nimodipine for prophylaxis of cerebral vasospasm in aneurysmal subarachnoid haemorrhage (BRANT trial)

The 'British Aneurysm Nimodipine Trial' was one of the first properly randomized trials involving neurosurgical patients. It showed reduced cerebral infarction and better outcome in patients given nimodipine. Pickard *et al.* published the "Effect of oral nimodipine on cerebral infarction and outcome after subarachnoid haemorrhage: British Aneurysm Nimodipine Trial" in *BMJ* in 1989.

In this trial, 60 mg of oral nimodipine was given 4 hourly and continued for 21 days. The outcome was observed whether nimodipine reduces the incidence of cerebral ischaemia and infarction arising de novo after spontaneous CT/LP proven aneurysmal SAH. The main distinction in outcome was between moderate or good outcome and poor outcome, i.e., death or severe disability.

Patients of <18 years, SAH older than 96 hours, patients having major comorbidities (renal, hepatic, pulmonary, cardiac disease); coma due to SAH within the week prior to latest SAH and lack of consent were excluded.

Follow-up results at 3 months showed that nimodipine treatment with the specified duration reduced the incidence of cerebral infarction by one-third (22% with nimodipine compared to 33% with placebo). There was a reduction of definite infarcts from 34% or 37%, which was statistically significant ($p = 0.014$). Poor outcomes reduced significantly by 40% with nimodipine compared to placebo (20% vs. 33%, respectively, $p < 0.001$). There was no significant effect on mortality between the groups.

The authors concluded that 60 mg of oral nimodipine 4 hourly is well tolerated and reduces cerebral infarction and improves outcome after SAH. Based on this study, it is now almost a worldwide practice to give nimodipine to all patients with SAH.

Study reference

Pickard JD, Murray GD, Illingworth R, Shaw MDM, Teasdale GM, Foy PM, Humphrey PRD, Lang DA, Nelson R, Richards P, Sinar J, Bailey S, Skene A. Effect of oral nimodipine on cerebral infarction and outcome after subarachnoid haemorrhage: British Aneurysm Nimodipine Trial. *BMJ* 1989; 298: 636–642.

Benefit of other calcium channel blockers In SAH

Dorhout Mees *et al.* published a systematic review of 27 randomized controlled trials (RCTs) in Cochrane Database Systematic Review in 2007, in which other calcium antagonists, such as nicardipine, have been investigated. In that review, there was the only evidence to support the prophylactic use of nimodipine (Mees *et al.*, 2007).

Study reference

Dorhout Mees SM, Rinkel GJE, Feigin VL, Algra A, van den Bergh WM, Vermeulen M, van Gijn N. Calcium antagonists for subarachnoid haemorrhage. *Cochrane Database Syst Rev* 2007; 3: CD000277

STASH trial

Kirkpatrick *et al.* conducted "Simvastatin in Acute Subarachnoid Haemorrhage (STASH) trial" which is an international, multicentre, parallel group, double-blind, randomized phase 3 trial, which was published in *Lancet Neurology* in 2014. The authors concluded that the trial did not detect any benefit in the use of simvastatin for long-term or short-term outcome in patients with aneurysmal SAH. Therefore, patients with SAH should not be treated routinely with simvastatin during the acute stages.

Study reference

Kirkpatrick PJ, Turner CL, Smith C, Hutchinson PJ, Murray GD; STASH Collaborators. Simvastatin in aneurysmal subarachnoid haemorrhage (STASH): a multicentre randomised phase 3 trial. *Lancet Neurol* 2014 Jul; *13(7)*: 666–675. DOI: 10.1016/S1474-4422(14)70084-5. Epub 2014 May 15. PMID: 24837690.

ARUBA trial

Mohr *et al.* conducted this multicentre, non-blinded, randomized trial to compare the outcome of medical management with interventional therapy which included neurosurgery, embolization or stereotactic radiotherapy, alone or in combination or medical management alone for unruptured brain arteriovenous malformations (ARUBA). Adult patients (≥18 years) with an unruptured brain arteriovenous malformation were enroled into this trial at 39 clinical sites in nine countries.

The result showed that medical management is superior as the risk of death or stroke was significantly lower in the medical management group than in the interventional therapy group. Interventional therapy group showed a higher number of strokes (45 vs. 12, $p < 0.0001$) and neurological deficits unrelated to stroke (14 vs. 1, $p = 0.0008$) when compared with the medical management group.

The authors concluded that medical management alone is superior to medical management with interventional therapy for the prevention of death or stroke in patients with unruptured brain arteriovenous malformations followed up for 33 months.

This trial became an object of comments and criticisms following its publication. The frequently mentioned concerns were the design of the study, with heterogeneity of patients and the lack of standardization of the treatment arm. The choice of outcome measures was repeatedly criticized. During the trial, low enrolment rates, selection bias and premature interruption of enrolment were frequent comments. The short follow-up period, the lack of subgroup analyses, the lack of details on the results of the various treatments and a contentious interpretation of results were noted at the analysis stage.

Study reference

Mohr JP, Parides MK, Stapf C, Moquete E, Moy CS, Overbey JR, Al-Shahi Salman R, Vicaut E, Young WL, Houdart E, Cordonnier C, Stefani MA, Hartmann A, von Kummer R, Biondi A, Berkefeld J, Klijn CJ, Harkness K, Libman R, Barreau X, Moskowitz AJ; International ARUBA Investigators. Medical management with or without interventional therapy for unruptured brain arteriovenous malformations (ARUBA): a multicentre, non-blinded, randomised trial. *Lancet* 2014 Feb 15; *383(9917)*: 614–621. DOI: 10.1016/S0140-6736(13)62302-8. Epub 2013 Nov 20. PMID: 24268105; PMCID: PMC4119885.

Other important publications from vascular neurosurgery

Allen GS, Ahn HS, Preziosi TJ, *et al.* Cerebral arterial spasm – a controlled trial of nimodipine in patients with subarachnoid hemorrhage. *N Engl J Med* 1983; *308(11)*: 619–624.

Awad IA, Carter LP, Spetzler RF, *et al.* Clinical vasospasm after subarachnoid hemorrhage: response to hypervolemic hemodilution and arterial hypertension. *Stroke* 1987; *18(2)*: 365–372.

Barrow DL, Spector RH, Braun IF, *et al.* Classification and treatment of spontaneous carotid-cavernous fistulas. *J Neurosurg* 1985; *62*: 248–256.

Biljenga P, Gondar R, Schilling S. PHASES score for the management of intracranial aneurysm. *Stroke* 2017; *48(8)*: 2105–2112.

Diringer MN, Bleck, TP, Hemphill JC, *et al.* Critical care management of patients following aneurysmal subarachnoid hemorrhage: recommendations from the Neurocritical Care Society's Multidisciplinary Consensus Conference. *Neurocrit Care* 2011; *15*: 211–240.

Fisher CM, Kistler JP, Davis JM. Relation of cerebral vasospasm to subarachnoid hemorrhage visualized by computerized tomographic scanning. *Neurosurgery* 1980; *6(1)*: 1–9.

Gobin YP, Laurent A, Merienne L, *et al.* Treatment of brain arteriovenous malformations by embolization and radiosurgery. *J Neurosurg* 1996; *85(1)*: 19–28.

Guglielmi G, Viñuela F, Dion, J, *et al.* Electrothrombosis of saccular aneurysms via endovascular approach. Part 2: Preliminary clinical experience. *J Neurosurg* 1991; *75(1)*: 8–14.

Juvela S, Porras M, Heiskanen O. Natural history of unruptured intracranial aneurysms: a long-term follow-up study. *J Neurosurg* 1993; *79(2)*: 174–182.

Mast H, Young WL, Koennecke HC, *et al.* Risk of spontaneous haemorrhage after diagnosis of cerebral arteriovenous malformation. *Lancet* 1997; *350(9084)*: 1065–1068.

McDougall CG, Spetzler RF, Zabramski JM, *et al.* The Barrow Ruptured Aneurysm Trial. *J Neurosurg* 2012; *116(1)*: 135–144.

Solenski NJ, Haley EC Jr, Kassell NF, *et al.* Medical complications of aneurysmal subarachnoid hemorrhage: a report of the Multicenter, Cooperative Aneurysm Study. Participants of the Multicenter Cooperative Aneurysm Study. *Crit Care Med* 1995; *23(6)*: 1007–1017.

Spetzler RF, Martin NA. A proposed grading system for arteriovenous malformations. *J Neurosurg* 1986; *65(4)*: 476–483.

Spetzler RF, Ponce FA. A 3-tier classification of cerebral arteriovenous malformations. *J Neurosurg* 2011; *114(3)*: 842–849.

Cranial trauma

Decompressive craniectomy for severe traumatic brain injury

Decompressive craniectomy (DC) was a widely accepted surgical method when medical treatment fails to control high intracranial pressure (ICP) in patients with severe traumatic brain injury (TBI) based on results from non-randomized trials and a few controlled trials with historical control.

Decompressive Craniectomy (DECRA) trial

DECRA is the first well-designed, multi-centre RCT, which reviewed the role of DC in severe TBI. Cooper DJ *et al.* carried out DECRA study on "Craniectomy plus standard care versus standard care alone" in 15 centres of Australia, New Zealand and Saudi Arabia from 2002 to 2010, published in the *New England Journal of Medicine* in 2011.

In this trial, patients were randomized within 72 hours of injury to DC and standard care vs. standard care alone. Standard care included all the recommended methods of controlling ICP like sedation, normalization of arterial PCO_2, mannitol or hypertonic saline, neuromuscular blockade, external ventricular drainage as first tier and mild hypothermia and barbiturate as second tier as suggested by Brain Trauma Foundation (BTF) guidelines. Decompressive craniectomy consisted of a bifrontal craniectomy with bilateral dural opening, while the falx and sagittal sinus were preserved.

Patients of 15–59 years, with severe, non-penetrating head injury (GCS 3–8), were included following informed consent from the next of kin. Patients with fixed dilated pupils; mass lesion; spinal cord injury and pre-hospital cardiac arrest were excluded. All patients were admitted in advance neuro-ITU with ICP monitoring. Refractory ICP was defined as persistently raised ICP>20 mmHg for >15 minutes within a 1-hours period.

The craniectomy group had a worse Extended Glasgow Outcome Score than those receiving standard care alone ($p = 0.03$). There was also a greater risk of unfavourable outcome ($p = 0.02$) in the craniectomy group. Hydrocephalus was also found to be tenfold more in the craniectomy group (10%) than in the standard-care group (1%). It seemed that any potential improvement in controlling ICP obtained by surgical decompression may well be offset by surgical morbidity. The authors speculated that the expansion of the brain outside the skull vault may have resulted in axonal stretch injury, which eventually caused the harmful effects of DC.

It was concluded that in adults with severe diffuse TBI and refractory intracranial hypertension, early DC was effective in reducing ICP and length of ICU stay, but it was associated with more unfavourable outcomes for adult patients with severe TBI.

Study reference
Cooper DJ, Rosenfeld JV, Murray L, Arabi YM, Davies AR, D'Urso P, Kossmann T, Ponsford J, Seppelt I, Reilly P, Wolfe R. Decompressive craniectomy in diffuse traumatic brain injury. N Engl J Med 2011; 364: 1493–1502.

Randomized Evaluation of Surgery with Craniectomy for Uncontrollable Elevation of intracranial pressure (RESCUEicp) trial

Hutchinson et al. carried out a study to assess the effectiveness of craniectomy as a last-tier intervention in patients with TBI and refractory intracranial hypertension in 52 centres in 20 countries from January 2004 to March 2014. The result was published in the NEJM in 2016.

Patients aged between 10 and 65 years were treated in ICUs to maintain an ICP of 25 mmHg or less by stepwise treatment. Patients with bilateral fixed and dilated pupils, bleeding diathesis, or with an unsurvivable injury were excluded.

Stage 1 included sedation, analgesia and head elevation; neuromuscular blockade (optional). Other targets included a CPP of more than 60 mmHg, normothermia, normoglycemia, mild hypocapnia and adequate oxygenation (O_2 saturation >97%).

If ICP was not controlled, stage 2 options included ventricular drain, pharmacologic blood-pressure augmentation, osmotherapy, moderate hypocapnia and therapeutic hypothermia.

If ICP remained above 25 mmHg for 1–12 hours despite these measures, then at stage 3 of the protocol, patients were randomly assigned to undergo DC (either large unilateral hemicraniectomy for patients with unilateral hemispheric swelling or bifrontal craniectomy for patients with diffuse brain swelling) with medical therapy or to receive continued medical therapy with the option of adding barbiturates to reduce ICP.

The study reveals that death rate is much lower in patients who underwent DC (26.9% at 6 months) than in those who received medical therapies only (48.9%). However, the survivors were far more likely to end up with poor neurological outcomes (vegetative state or with lower severe disability) at both 6 and 12 months.

There are a few noteworthy differences between DECRA and RESCUEicp. First, the ICP threshold for intervention was lower in DECRA (20 mmHg) than in RESCUEicp (25 mmHg). RESCUEicp had a more permissive approach allowing ICP >25 mmHg for 1–12 hours. On the other hand, DECRA aimed to evaluate the effects of early decompression, intervening at an ICP >20 mmHg for more than 15 minutes.

Only bifrontal craniectomies were allowed in DECRA as the decompressive surgery. In RESCUEicp, leaving the surgical options on the discretion of the treating surgeons, bifrontal craniectomy was lower at 63%; the rest was unilateral hemicraniectomies.

Furthermore, a significant proportion of patients (37%) randomized to the medical arm of RESCUEicp ended up with a "rescue" craniectomy. These were performed in cases where other measures were exhausted, and the managing medical team deemed it reasonable.

Study reference

Hutchinson PJ, Kolias AG, Timofeev IS, Corteen EA, Czosnyka M, Timothy J, Anderson I, Bulters DO, Belli A, Eynon CA, Wadley J, Mendelow AD, Mitchell PM, Wilson MH, Critchley G, Sahuquillo J, Unterberg A, Servadei F, Teasdale GM, Pickard JD, Menon DK, Murray GD, Kirkpatrick PJ; RESCUEicp Trial Collaborators. Trial of decompressive craniectomy for traumatic intracranial hypertension. N Engl J Med. 2016 Sep 22; 375(12): 1119–30. DOI: 10.1056/NEJMoa1605215. Epub 2016 Sep 7. PMID: 27602507.

Surgical Trial in Traumatic Intracerebral Haemorrhage (STITCH)

Gregson et al. conducted this study to evaluate the results of early surgery within 12 hours and Initial Conservative Treatment with delayed evacuation if it became clinically appropriate. It was carried out in neurosurgical units in 59 hospitals in 20 countries.

Patients in the Early Surgery group were 10.5% more likely to have a favourable outcome (absolute benefit), but this difference did not quite reach statistical significance because of the reduced sample size. Mortality was significantly higher in the Initial Conservative Treatment group (33% vs. 15%).

The authors concluded that early surgery may be a valuable tool in the treatment of TICH, especially if the GCS is between 9 and 12, as was also found in previous STICH trials for spontaneous intracerebral haematoma.

Study reference

Gregson BA, Rowan EN, Francis R, McNamee P, Boyers D, Mitchell P, McColl E, Chambers IR, Unterberg A, Mendelow AD; STITCH(TRAUMA) Investigators. Surgical Trial In Traumatic intraCerebral Haemorrhage (STITCH): a randomised controlled trial of Early Surgery compared with Initial Conservative Treatment. Health Technol Assess 2015 Sep; 19(70): 1–138. DOI: 10.3310/hta19700. PMID: 26346805; PMCID: PMC4780887.

Timing of surgery for acute traumatic extra-axial haematomas

Mendelow *et al.* studied the delay between neurological deterioration and surgery and the outcome of and published "Extradural haematomas: effect of delayed treatment" in *BMJ* in 1979. In this study, when patients were routinely admitted directly to the neurosurgical unit within 24 hours that resulted in a fourfold reduction in a delay to surgery. The mean duration of delay to surgery in survivors was 1.9 hours and that in non-survivors was 15.7 hours. The difference was statistically significant ($p < 0.05$).

Seelig *et al.* published "Traumatic acute subdural hematoma: major mortality reduction in comatose patients treated within four hours" in *JAMA* in 1981. In this series, those patients were included who had acute subdural haematoma causing >5 mm midline shift, neurological status: impaired verbal response (unable to speak in response to noxious stimuli); unresponsive to verbal command, negative drug/alcohol screen and spontaneous respiration.

This study defines the delay as time from injury to surgery. The patients who were operated <4 hours from injury had 30% mortality, and those who were operated >4 hours from injury had 90% mortality. The difference was statistically significant ($p < 0.0001$).

Seelig *et al.* also found poor pre-operative neurological status led to increased mortality ($p < 0.05$) and post-operative control of ICP <20 mmHg was associated with functional recovery in 79% of patients ($p < 0.001$).

Study reference

Seelig JM, Becker DP, Miller JD, Greenberg RP, Ward JD, Choi SC. Traumatic acute subdural hematoma: major mortality reduction in comatose patients treated within four hours. *JAMA* 1981; *304*: 1511–1518

Surgery for chronic subdural haematomas (CSDH)

Drain vs. no drain

Santarius *et al.* published "Use of drains versus no drains after burr-hole evacuation of chronic subdural haematoma: a randomized controlled trial" in *Lancet* in 2009. This RCT was carried out at Addenbrooke's Hospital in Cambridge, UK, between 2004 and 2007 to address the role of drains following burr-hole drainage of CSDH.

Two hundred fifteen patients were included who were >18 years and had symptomatic CT confirmed CSDH. Those cases of CSDH who had surgery other than burr-hole evacuation, ipsilateral CSF shunt insertion within the preceding 6 months and drain placement were thought to be unsafe. The rate of recurrence with a drain was 9.3% and without drain was 24%. With this statistically significant ($p = 0.003$) difference, the trial was stopped early.

At discharge, patients with drains were reported to have fewer neurological deficits, a better functional status and more favourable modified Rankin scores. However, there were no significant differences in complication rates between the two groups.

The authors concluded that the use of a drain after burr-hole drainage of chronic subdural haematoma is safe and associated with reduced recurrence and mortality at 6 months.

Study reference

Santarius T, Kirkpatrick PJ, Ganesan D, Chia HL, Jalloh I, Smielewski P, Richards HK, Marcus H, Parker RA, Price SJ, Kirollos RW, Pickard JD, Hutchinson PJ. Use of drains versus no drains after burr-hole evacuation of chronic subdural haematoma: a randomised controlled trial. *Lancet* 2009 Sep 26; *374(9695)*: 1067–73. DOI: 10.1016/S0140-6736(09)61115-6. PMID: 19782872.

Steroids in TBI

The Corticosteroids Randomization After Significant Head Injury (CRASH) trial is the largest multi-centre, international RCT looking at the effect of methylprednisolone on the risk of death and disability after head injury. CRASH trial collaborators published "Effects of intravenous corticosteroids on death within 14 days in 10008 adults with clinically significant head injury (MRC CRASH trial)" in *Lancet* in 2004. The collaborators also published "Final results of MRC CRASH, a randomized placebo-controlled trial of intravenous corticosteroid in adults with head injury—outcomes at 6 months" in *Lancet* in 2005.

In this trial, methylprednisolone infusion was studied against placebo. Methylprednisolone was administered within 8 hours of injury with a loading dose of 2 g (in 100 mL) over an hour period followed by the maintenance dose for 48 hours.

In the methylprednisolone group, the rate of death in 2 weeks (21.1%) and in 6 months (25.7%) was higher than the rate in 2 weeks (17.9%) and in 6 months (22.3%) in the placebo group, and the difference was statistically significant ($p < 0.001$). There was no statistically significant disability at 6 months.

The authors concluded that steroids should not be routinely used in the treatment of the head injury.

Study reference

Edwards P, Arango M, Balica L, Cottingham R, El-Sayed H, Farrell B, Fernandes J, Gogichaisvili T, Golden N, Hartzenberg B, Husain M, Ulloa MI, Jerbi Z, Khamis H, Komolafe E, Laloë V, Lomas G, Ludwig S, Mazairac G, Muñoz Sanchéz Mde L, Nasi L, Olldashi F, Plunkett P, Roberts I, Sandercock P, Shakur H, Soler C, Stocker R, Svoboda P, Trenkler S, Venkataramana NK, Wasserberg J, Yates D, Yutthakasemsunt S; CRASH Trial Collaborators. Final results of MRC CRASH, a randomised placebo-controlled trial of intravenous corticosteroid in adults with head injury-outcomes at 6 months. *Lancet* 2005 Jun 4–10; *365(9475)*: 1957–1959. DOI: 10.1016/S0140-6736(05)66552-X. PMID: 15936423.

Barbiturates in TBI

Eisenberg *et al.* published "High-dose barbiturates control elevated ICP in patients with severe head injury" in *Journal of Neurosurgery* in 1988. This is the first RCT to assess the efficacy of pentobarbital over the best conventional therapy to treat elevated ICP in severely head-injured patients. The trial was carried out from 1982 to 1987 in the United States.

The patients of 15–50 years were included having GCS 4–7 post-resuscitation, serum osmolality ≥315 mOsm/kg; mannitol was given within 1 hours prior to randomisation. The patients with GCS 3, fixed pupils or pregnancy were excluded.

Multiple logistic model statistical analysis revealed a significant positive treatment effect of pentobarbital ($p = 0.04$). Uncontrolled ICP was robustly associated with death in both treatment arms. On the other hand, >90% of patients with controlled ICP survived.

The authors concluded that high-dose barbiturates are an appropriate adjunct in the control of raised ICP in severely head-injured patients.

Study reference

Eisenberg HM, Frankowski RF, Contant CF, Marshall LF, Walker MD. High-dose barbiturates control elevated intracranial pressure in patients with severe head injury. *J Neurosurg* 1988; 69: 15–23.

Hyperosmolar therapy to control raised ICP in TBI

Cruz *et al.* published their finding on three different cohorts of patients on neurosurgery in 2001, 2002 and 2004. Those three cohorts included patients with subdural haematomas (ASDH), temporal intraparenchymal haematomas (IPH) and diffuse brain injury (DBI). Early administration of high-dose mannitol leads to significant improvements and better clinical outcomes in patients with ASDH, traumatic temporal IPH and DBI.

Study references

Cruz J, Minoja G, Okuchi K. Improving clinical outcomes from acute subdural hematomas with the emergency *preoperative* administration of high doses of mannitol: a randomized trial. *Neurosurgery* 2001; 49: 864–871.
Cruz J, Minoja G, Okuchi K. Major clinical and physiological benefits of early high doses of mannitol for intraparenchymal temporal lobe hemorrhages with abnormal pupillary widening: a randomised trial. *Neurosurgery* 2002; 51: 628–637.
Cruz J, Minoja G, Okuchi K, Facco E. Successful use of the new high-dose mannitol treatment in patients with Glasgow Coma Scale scores of 3 and bilateral abnormal pupillary widening: a randomized trial. *Neurosurgery* 2004; 100: 376–383.

Hypertonic saline vs. mannitol

Vialet *et al.* published "Isovolume hypertonic solutes (sodium chloride or mannitol) in the treatment of refractory posttraumatic intracranial hypertension: 2 mgL/kg 7.5% saline is more effective than 2 mL/kg 20% mannitol" in *Critical Care Medicine* in 2003. Between the Hypertonic Saline (HS) group and the Mannitol group, the mean number of episodes of raised ICP/day and the duration of episodes of raised ICP/day were significantly lower in the HS group ($p < .01$). The rate of clinical failure (which was defined as failure to reduce ICP <25 mmHg or to increase cerebral perfusion pressure (CPP) to over 70 mmHg after two sequential boluses of hypertonic fluid) was also significantly lower ($p < .01$) in the HS group. There was no significant difference in mortality or Glasgow outcome score (GOS) between the two treatment arms. Hence, it was concluded that HS is an effective and safe initial treatment for intracranial hypertension episodes in TBI patients when osmotherapy is needed.

Study reference

Vialet R, Albanese J, Thomachot L, Antonini R, Bourgouin A, Alliez B, Martin C. Isovolume hypertonic solutes (sodium chloride or mannitol) in the treatment of refractory posttraumatic intracranial hypertension: 2 mgL/kg 7.5% saline is more effective than 2 mL/kg 20% mannitol. *Crit Care Med* 2003; *31*: 1683–1687.

Hypothermia in TBI

The role of therapeutic hypothermia in severe TBI was assessed through a number of single-centre trials. Clifton *et al.* carried out the first multi-centre randomized trial of treatment with hypothermia for patients with severe TBI as the National Acute Brain Injury Study: Hypothermia (NABIS: H I) in the United States between 1994 and 1998 and published "Lack of effect of induction of hypothermia after acute brain injury" in the *New England Journal of Medicine* in 2001. NABIS: H I aimed to determine the efficacy of therapeutic hypothermia within 8 hours of injury.

Clifton *et al.* also carried out the second multi-centre randomized trial which was the National Acute Brain Injury Study: Hypothermia (NABIS: H II) in the United States and Canada between 2005 and 2009. NABIS: H II aimed to assess the efficacy of very early therapeutic hypothermia within 2.5 hours of injury. This was published in *Lancet* in 2011.

From the results, the authors concluded from both NABIS: H I and NABIS: H II that hypothermic treatment following severe TBI does not improve functional outcome.

Study references

Clifton GL, Miller ER, Choi SC, Levin HS, McCauley S, Smith K, Muizelaar JP, Wagner FC, Marion DW, Luerssen TG, Chestnut RM, Schwartz M. Lack of effect of induction of hypothermia after acute brain injury. *N Engl J Med* 2001; *344*: 556–563.

Clifton GL, Valadka, Zygun D, Coffey CS, Drever P, Fourwinds S, Janis LS, Wilde E, Taylor P, Harshman K, Conley A, Puccio A, Levin HS, McCauley SR, Bucholz RD, Smith KR, Schmidy JH, Scott JN, Yonas H, Okonkwo DO. Very early hypothermia induction in patients with severe brain injury (the National Acute Brain Injury Study: Hypothermia II): a randomised trial. *Lancet* 2011; *10*: 131–139.

Hyperventilation in head injury

Muizelaar *et al.* carried out the only randomized trial at the Medical College of Virginia evaluating the role of hyperventilation on outcome in severe TBI and published "Adverse effects of prolonged hyperventilation in patients with severe traumatic brain injury" in *Journal of Neurosurgery* in 1991.

This trial has been the most influential study to date. It compared normoventilation, hyperventilation and hyperventilation plus tromomethamine (THAM). The authors concluded that prophylactic hyperventilation is deleterious in TBI patients who presented with a motor score of 4–5.

Study reference

Muizelaar JP, Marmarou A, Ward JD, Kontos HA, Choi SC, Becker DP, Gruemer H, Young HF. Adverse effects of prolonged hyperventilation in patients with severe traumatic brain injury. *J Neurosurg* 1991; 75: 731–739.

Post-traumatic seizures (PTS) in TBI

Annegers *et al.* carried out a study on 4541 people who had TBI from 1935 to 1984 in Minnesota, United States and published "A population-based study of seizures after traumatic brain injuries" in the *New England Journal of Medicine* in 1998.

This study found there was no increased risk of seizures for mild TBI after 5 years, but with moderate TBI, there is a significantly increased risk of seizures for over 10 years, and with severe TBI, there is a significantly increased risk of seizures for over 20 years. Cumulative 5-year probability of seizure from mild TBI is 0.7%, moderate TBI is 1.2 and severe TBI is 10%. Brain contusions and subdural haematomas were identified as the strongest risk factors for PTS. Skull fracture and prolonged loss of consciousness also bear risks of PTS.

Christensen *et al.* carried out a large population-based study on 78,572 people with TBI born from 1977 to 2002 using the Civil Registration System in Denmark and published "Long-term risk of epilepsy after traumatic brain injury in children and young adults: a population-based cohort study" in *Lancet* in 2009.

The results of this study showed the relative risk (RR) of epilepsy increased with age, and RR of PTS was more in women (2.49) than in men (2.01). In patients >15 years of age at time of injury, RR was 3.51 for mild and 12.24 for a severe head injury. RR of epilepsy was also increased in those with a family history of epilepsy (5.75 mild and 10.09 severe head injury). The authors also concluded traumatic head injury is a long-lasting risk factor for epilepsy, and there is a window for prevention of post-traumatic epilepsy.

NB: Definitions of mild and severe brain injury were according to the American Congress of Rehabilitation Medicine: Mild brain injury is manifest by altered brain function (loss of consciousness <30 minutes, GCS not <13, amnesia <24 hours, confusion); severe brain injury includes contusion and intracranial haemorrhage.

Study references

Annegers JF, Hauser WA, Coan SP, Rocca WA. A population-based study of seizures after traumatic brain injuries. *N Engl J Med* 1998; 338: 20–24.
Christensen J, Pedersen MG, Pedersen CB, Sidenius P, Olsen J, Vestergaard M. Long-term risk of epilepsy after traumatic brain injury in children and young adults: a population-based cohort study. *Lancet* 2009; 373: 1105–1110.

Phenytoin for prevention of PTS

Temkin *et al.* carried out the first PRCT in the mid-1980s at the Harborview Medical Center, Washington, United States to evaluate the efficacy of phenytoin for the prophylaxis of PTS following severe TBI and published "A randomised, double-blind study of phenytoin for the prevention of post-traumatic seizures" in the *New England Journal of Medicine* in 1990.

Patients were included if: presence of a severe TBI defined as one or more of CT proven cortical contusion; EDH; SDH; ICH; depressed skull fracture; penetrating head injury; seizure <24 hours from injury and GCS ≤10.

Patients, who were younger than 16 years or with predisposing risk factors for seizures, e.g. previous severe head injury, history of severe alcoholism or previous neurological conditions with risk of seizures or if there was a delay of >24 hours before loading of a drug, were excluded.

The initial loading dose of phenytoin was 20 mg/kg with the maintenance dose adjusted according to serum levels. Phenytoin/placebo was continued for 12 months and was then tapered off fully.

The authors concluded that only in the first week following severe TBI, phenytoin has a beneficial effect in reducing the incidence of PTS.

Study reference

Temkin NR, Dikmen SS, Wilensky AJ, Keihm J, Chabal S, Winn HR. A randomised, double-blind study of phenytoin for the prevention of post-traumatic seizures. *N Engl J Med* 1990; 323: 497–502.

Intracranial pressure monitoring in TBI

Guillaume and Hanny (1951) and Lundberg (1960) were the pioneers to introduce ICP monitoring into neurosurgical practice. Studies by Miller *et al.* in 1977 and 1981 firmly established the importance of ICP monitoring for the standard care of TBI.

In 2012, Chestnut *et al.* published "A trial of intracranial-pressure monitoring in traumatic brain injury" in the *New England Journal of Medicine*. This is also known as BEST:TRIP trial (Benchmark Evidence from South American Trials: Treatment of Intracranial Pressure trial) from centres in Bolivia and Ecuador, a landmark trial of ICP monitoring in TBI. Despite the established importance of ICP monitoring, the investigators could overcome the ethical barrier by carrying out this trial in intensive care units where, because of local doubts about the efficacy, the ICP monitoring was not routinely used.

In this trial, patients of more than 13 years, with GCS 3–8 (M ≤ 5 if intubated) within 48 hours of injury were included. Patients with bilateral fixed and dilated pupils were excluded. An intraparenchymal ICP monitor was placed and ICP was maintained <20 mmHg in accordance with the BTF/American Association of Neurological Surgeons guidelines. The other group of TBI was treated based on imaging and clinical examination.

There was no significant difference between the two groups in the primary outcome, i.e., survival time, impaired consciousness, functional status and neuropsychological status. There were no differences in 6-month mortality between the two groups: 41% in the ICP monitored group compared to 39% in the imaging-clinical examination group ($p = 0.60$).

Hutchinson *et al.* from the Cambridge Head Injury Group have published their evaluation of the BEST:TRIP trial and argue that there should be no fundamental change in the management of severe TBI. Non-conventional use of a composite outcome measure was also criticized by the Cambridge head injury group. They observed that if the more conventional GOS was used, then mortality and favourable outcome favoured the ICP monitoring arm, although the difference was small (5%) and non-significant.

Study reference

Chestnut RM, Temkin N, Carney N, Dikmen S, Rondina C, Videtta W, Petroni G, Pridgeon J, Barber J, Machamer J, Chaddock K, Celix K, Cherner M, Hendrix T. A trial of intracranial-pressure monitoring in traumatic brain injury. *N Engl J Med* 2012; 367: 2471–2481.

Dexamethasone for Chronic Subdural Hematoma (DEX-CSDH) trial

Hutchinson *et al.* conducted a multi-centre, randomized trial in the UK to study the effect of dexamethasone on adult patients with symptomatic CSDH. The result was published in the *New England Journal of Medicine* in 2020. The study population received a 2-week tapering course of oral dexamethasone, starting at 8 mg twice daily, or placebo. The decision to surgically evacuate the hematoma was made by the treating clinician. The authors concluded that among adults with symptomatic CSDH, treatment with dexamethasone following the evacuation of CSDH during the index admission resulted in fewer favourable outcomes and more adverse events than placebo at 6 months, but fewer repeat operations were performed in the dexamethasone group.

Study reference

Kolias AG, Edlmann E, Thelin EP, Bulters D, Holton P, Suttner N, Owusu-Agyemang K, Al-Tamimi YZ, Gatt D, Thomson S, Anderson IA, Richards O, Whitfield P, Gherle M, Caldwell K, Davis-Wilkie C, Tarantino S, Barton G, Marcus HJ, Chari A, Brennan P, Belli A, Bond S, Turner C, Whitehead L, Wilkinson I, Hutchinson PJ; British Neurosurgical Trainee Research Collaborative (BNTRC) and Dex-CSDH Trial Collaborators. Dexamethasone for adult patients with a symptomatic chronic subdural haematoma (Dex-CSDH) trial: study protocol for a randomised controlled trial. *Trials* 2018 Dec 4; *19(1)*: 670. DOI: 10.1186/s13063-018-3050-4. Erratum in: Trials. 2019 Mar 18; *20(1)*: 175. Zolnouria, Ardalan [corrected to Zolnourian, Ardalan]. PMID: 30514400; PMCID: PMC6280536.

CRASH 2 trial

CRASH 2 is not a neurosurgical trial. But, as the link between the CRASH and CRASH 3 trial, this is briefly discussed here.

CRASH-2 trial collaborators published a study on "Effects of tranexamic acid (TXA) on death, vascular occlusive events, and blood transfusion in trauma patients with significant haemorrhage (CRASH-2): a randomised, placebo-controlled trial" in *Lancet* in 2010.

Patients >18 years with trauma, presented within 8 hours of incident with either significant haemorrhage or at the risk of significant haemorrhage, were included. They were given a loading dose of 1 g of TXA over 10 minutes, followed by an intravenous infusion of 1 g over 8 hours.

The authors concluded that TXA safely reduced the risk of death in bleeding trauma patients in this study. On the basis of these results, TXA should be considered for use in bleeding trauma patients.

Study reference

Roberts I, Shakur H, Coats T, Hunt B, Balogun E, Barnetson L, Cook L, Kawahara T, Perel P, Prieto-Merino D, Ramos M, Cairns J, Guerriero C. The CRASH-2 Trial: a randomised controlled trial and economic evaluation of the effects of tranexamic acid on death, vascular occlusive events and transfusion requirement in bleeding trauma patients. *Health Technol Assess* 2013 Mar; *17(10)*: 1–79. DOI: 10.3310/hta17100. PMID: 23477634; PMCID: PMC4780956.

CRASH-3 trial

The CRASH-3 trial collaborators studied whether administration of TXA under 3 ho from injury, compared with placebo, reduce head injury associated in-hospital mortality within 28 days and published "Effects of tranexamic acid on death, disability, vascular occlusive events and other morbidities in patients with acute traumatic brain injury (CRASH-3): a randomised, placebo-controlled trial" in *Lancet* in 2019.

Inclusion criteria were the adult patients with TBI within 3 hours of injury (changed from within 8 hours of injury in Sep 2016), GCS ≤12 or intracranial bleeding on CT, no major external bleeding and the treating clinician was uncertain about the benefit of TXA as the treatment. TXA was given as 1 g over 10 minutes followed by intravenous infusion of 1 g over 8 hours.

Twenty-eight days in hospital TBI-associated mortality in the TXA group was significantly reduced in patients with mild to moderate TBI (GCS 9–15). The result also showed that early treatment was more effective than later treatment in mild to moderate injury ($p = 0.005$), but timing had no effect on severe injury.

The authors concluded that TXA is safe in TBI and that treatment within 3 hours reduces head injury-associated deaths.

Study reference

CRASH-3 Trial Collaborators. Effects of tranexamic acid on death, disability, vascular occlusive events and other morbidities in patients with acute traumatic brain injury (CRASH-3): a randomised, placebo-controlled trial. *Lancet* 2019 Nov 9; *394(10210)*: 1713–1723. DOI: 10.1016/S0140-6736(19)32233-0. Epub 2019 Oct 14. Erratum in: *Lancet*. 2019 Nov 9;394(10210):1712. PMID: 31623894; PMCID: PMC6853170.

Other important publications from neurosurgical trauma

Bouma GJ, Muizelaar JP, Bandoh K, *et al*. Blood pressure and intracranial pressure-volume dynamics in severe head injury: relationship with cerebral blood flow. *J Neurosurg* 1992; *77(1)*: 15–19.

Chesnut RM, Marshall LF, Klauber MR, *et al*. The role of secondary brain injury in determining outcome from severe head injury. *J Trauma* 1993; *34(2)*: 216–222.

Guerra WK, Gaab MR, Dietz H, *et al*. Surgical decompression for traumatic brain swelling: indications and results. *J Neurosurg* 1999; *90(2)*: 187–196.

Jennett B, Bond M. Assessment of outcome after severe brain damage. *Lancet* 1975; *1(7905)*: 480–484.

Marmarou A, Anderson RL, Ward JD. Impact of ICP instability and hypotension on outcome in patients with severe head trauma. *J Neurosurg* 1991; *75*: S59–S66.

Maynard FM Jr, Bracken MB, Creasey G, *et al*. International Standards for Neurological and Functional Classification of Spinal Cord Injury. American Spinal Injury Association. *Spinal Cord* 1997; *35(5)*: 266–274.

Murray GD, Teasdale GM, Braakman R, *et al*. The European Brain Injury Consortium survey of head injuries. *Acta Neurochir* 1999; *141(3)*: 223–236.

Polin RS, Shaffrey ME, Bogaev CA, *et al*. Decompressive bifrontal craniectomy in the treatment of severe refractory post-traumatic cerebral edema. *Neurosurgery* 1997; *41(1)*: 84–92; discussion 92–94.

Roberts I, Yates D, Sandercock P, *et al*. Effect of intravenous corticosteroids on death within 14 days in 10 008 adults with clinically significant head injury (MRC CRASH trial): randomised placebo-controlled trial. *Lancet* 2004; *364(9442)*: 1321–1328.

Rosner MJ, Rosner SD, Johnson AH. Cerebral perfusion pressure: management protocol and clinical results. *J Neurosurg* 1995; *83(6)*: 949–962.

SAFE Study Investigators; Australian and New Zealand Intensive Care Society Clinical Trials Group, Australian Red Cross Blood Service, George Institute for International Health. Saline or albumin for fluid resuscitation in patients with traumatic brain injury. *N Engl J Med* 2007; *357(9)*: 874–884.

Teasdale G, Jennett B. Assessment of coma and impaired consciousness. A practical scale. *Lancet* 1974; *2(7872)*: 81–84.

Wilberger JE Jr, Harris M, Diamond DL. Acute subdural hematoma: morbidity, mortality, and operative timing. *J Neurosurg* 1991; *74(2)*: 212–218.

Stroke

Surgical intervention for spontaneous intracerebral haematoma

Mendelow *et al.* conducted study in 83 centres in 27 countries on "Early surgery versus initial conservative treatment in patients with spontaneous supratentorial intracerebral haematomas in the International Surgical Trial in Intracerebral Haemorrhage (STICH): a randomised trial", which was published in *Lancet* in 2005.

Surgery included craniotomy and CT-guided aspiration of the clot, and the method chosen was left to the discretion of the operating surgeon. The option of delayed surgery remained open to those who were randomized to the medical arm. Patients having CT evidence of intracerebral haematoma within 72 hours; clinical uncertainty regarding the benefits of either treatment arm of the trial; haematoma diameter >2 cm and GCS ≥5 were included.

Prognosis-based analyses did not reveal any statistically significant differences between the two arms of the trial. Subgroup analysis showed that a favourable outcome was more likely with early surgery for superficially based lesions (≤1 cm from the cortical surface) with a 29% relative benefit, but this difference was not statistically significant. It was concluded that there is no overall benefit from early surgery vs. initial conservative treatment for spontaneous supratentorial haematomas.

Unfortunately, STICH has been overinterpreted by some to mean that surgery does not have any beneficial role for supratentorial haematomas. However, STICH only looked at haematomas for which the responsible surgeon was not certain that surgery would help the patient more than the conservative management. The results of

STICH confirm that surgeons are correct to be uncertain about these patients, but the results cannot be extrapolated to all intracerebral haematomas.

Study reference

Mendelow AD, Gregson BA, Fernandes HM, Murray GD, Teasdale GM, Hope DT, Karimi A, Shaw MD, Barer DH; STICH Investigators. Early surgery versus initial conservative treatment in patients with spontaneous supratentorial intracerebral haematomas in the International Surgical Trial in Intracerebral Haemorrhage (STICH): a randomised trial. *Lancet* 2005 Jan 29–Feb 4; *365(9457)*: 387–397. DOI: 10.1016/S0140-6736(05)17826-X. PMID: 15680453.

STICH II trial

In STICH, the median time to perform surgery was 30 hours, which was relatively long after the presentation. Much earlier surgery, e.g. within 12 hours of the initial bleed, was thought to be of benefit. In addition, most patients underwent craniotomy (77%); hence, the role for more minimally invasive methods for evacuating haematomas came into question. Based on the subgroup analysis suggesting the benefit from early surgery in patients with superficial lobar haemorrhage, subsequent STICH II trial was conducted.

Mendelow *et al.* conducted "Early surgery versus initial conservative treatment in patients with spontaneous supratentorial lobar intracerebral haematomas (STICH II): a randomised trial" where Early surgery (12 hours from randomization) was compared with the best medical management and the result was published in *Lancet* in 2013. STICH II was a well-designed study along with excellent follow-up.

Surgery included craniotomy and CT-guided aspiration of the clot, and the method chosen was left to the discretion of the operating surgeon. Delayed surgery was allowed for those who were randomized to the medical arm.

Patients were included who had CT evidence of intracerebral lobar haematoma, superficial haematoma (up to 1 cm from surface of cortex, volume 10–100 mL) presented within 48 hours, clinical uncertainty regarding the benefits of either treatment arm of the trial, motor score 5 or 6; eye-opening score 2 or more (for confirmation of conscious at randomization).

Prognosis-based analyses did not reveal any statistically significant differences between the two arms of the trial. There was a survival advantage with no vegetative survivors at 6 months in the surgery group. But this was not statistically significant.

In the early surgery group, the mortality rate was 18% and unfavourable outcome 59%, while in the best medical management group, the mortality rate was 24% and unfavourable outcome was 62%. Nevertheless, it was not statistically significant. Hence, the authors concluded that there is no overall benefit from early surgery vs. initial conservative treatment for spontaneous superficial lobar supratentorial haematomas.

Study reference

Mendelow AD, Gregson BA, Rowan EN, Murray GD, Gholkar A, Mitchell PM; STICH II Investigators. Early surgery versus initial conservative treatment in patients with spontaneous supratentorial lobar intracerebral haematomas (STICH II): a randomised trial.

Lancet 2013 Aug 3; 382(9890): 397–408. DOI: 10.1016/S0140-6736(13)60986-1. Epub 2013 May 29. Erratum in: Lancet 2013 Aug 3; 382(9890): 396. Erratum in: Lancet 2021 Sep 18; 398(10305): 1042. PMID: 23726393; PMCID: PMC3906609.

Efficacy and safety of minimally invasive surgery with thrombolysis in intracerebral haemorrhage evacuation (MISTIE III): A randomized, controlled, open-label, blinded endpoint phase 3 trial

Hanley *et al.* conducted this study to assess whether minimally invasive catheter evacuation followed by thrombolysis (MISTIE), with the aim of decreasing clot size to 15 mL or less, would improve functional outcome in patients with intracerebral haemorrhage.

This was an open-label, blinded endpoint, phase 3 trial done at 78 hospitals in the United States, Canada, Europe, Australia and Asia. Patients aged 18 years or older with spontaneous, non-traumatic, supratentorial intracerebral haemorrhage of 30 mL or more were enroled. Patients randomized to image-guided MISTIE treatment for 1 mg alteplase 8 hourly for up to nine doses or standard medical care.

The authors concluded that for moderate to large intracerebral haemorrhage, MISTIE did not improve the proportion of patients who achieved a good response 365 days after intracerebral haemorrhage.

Study reference

Hanley DF, Thompson RE, Rosenblum M, Yenokyan G, Lane K, McBee N, Mayo SW, Bistran-Hall AJ, Gandhi D, Mould WA, Ullman N, Ali H, Carhuapoma JR, Kase CS, Lees KR, Dawson J, Wilson A, Betz JF, Sugar EA, Hao Y, Avadhani R, Caron JL, Harrigan MR, Carlson AP, Bulters D, LeDoux D, Huang J, Cobb C, Gupta G, Kitagawa R, Chicoine MR, Patel H, Dodd R, Camarata PJ, Wolfe S, Stadnik A, Money PL, Mitchell P, Sarabia R, Harnof S, Barzo P, Unterberg A, Teitelbaum JS, Wang W, Anderson CS, Mendelow AD, Gregson B, Janis S, Vespa P, Ziai W, Zuccarello M, Awad IA; MISTIE III Investigators. Efficacy and safety of minimally invasive surgery with thrombolysis in intracerebral haemorrhage evacuation (MISTIE III): a randomised, controlled, open-label, blinded endpoint phase 3 trial. Lancet 2019 Mar 9; 393(10175): 1021–1032. DOI: 10.1016/S0140-6736(19)30195-3. Epub 2019 Feb 7. Erratum in: Lancet 2019 Apr 20; 393(10181): 1596. PMID: 30739747; PMCID: PMC6894906.

CLEAR III trial

Hanley *et al.* published "Thrombolytic removal of intraventricular haemorrhage in treatment of severe stroke: results of the randomised, multicentre, multiregion, placebo-controlled CLEAR III trial" in *Lancet* in 2017.

In this trial (CLEAR III), in the ITU, patients with a routinely placed extraventricular drain (EVD), with stable, non-traumatic intracerebral haemorrhage volume less than 30 mL, intraventricular haemorrhage (IVH) obstructing the third or fourth ventricles and no underlying pathology were adaptively randomly assigned (1:1), to receive up to 12 doses, 8 hourly of 1 mg of alteplase or 0·9% saline via the EVD.

The authors concluded that in patients with IVH and a routine EVD, irrigation with alteplase did not substantially improve functional outcomes at the moderately severe disability (mRS) 3 cutoff compared with irrigation with saline. Protocol-based use of alteplase with EVD seems safe.

Study reference

Hanley DF, Lane K, McBee N, Ziai W, Tuhrim S, Lees KR, Dawson J, Gandhi D, Ullman N, Mould WA, Mayo SW, Mendelow AD, Gregson B, Butcher K, Vespa P, Wright DW, Kase CS, Carhuapoma JR, Keyl PM, Diener-West M, Muschelli J, Betz JF, Thompson CB, Sugar EA, Yenokyan G, Janis S, John S, Harnof S, Lopez GA, Aldrich EF, Harrigan MR, Ansari S, Jallo J, Caron JL, LeDoux D, Adeoye O, Zuccarello M, Adams HP Jr, Rosenblum M, Thompson RE, Awad IA; CLEAR III Investigators. Thrombolytic removal of intraventricular haemorrhage in treatment of severe stroke: results of the randomised, multicentre, multiregion, placebo-controlled CLEAR III trial. *Lancet* 2017 Feb 11; *389(10069)*: 603–611. DOI: 10.1016/S0140-6736(16)32410-2. Epub 2017 Jan 10. PMID: 28081952; PMCID: PMC6108339.

Decompressive surgery for malignant cerebral artery infarction

Malignant middle cerebral artery (MCA) infarction (MMI) is associated with a mortality rate of 80%. Since 2000, three European trials have addressed the role of decompressive surgery patients with MMI.

Vahedi *et al.* conducted the multicentre RCT named DECIMAL trial (DEcompressive Craniectomy In MALignant MCA infraction) performed in France which was published in *Stroke* in 2007. This trial was discontinued early because of recruitment problems, and a significant beneficial effect of surgery on mortality was found in an interim analysis.

Jüttler *et al.* conducted the multicentre RCT named DESTINY trial (DEcompressive Surgery for the Treatment of malignant Infarction of the MCA), which was performed in Germany and was published in *Stroke* in 2007. Similar to DECIMAL, recruitment to DESTINY was discontinued early because a predetermined analysis at 6 months showed a significant beneficial effect of surgery on mortality.

Hofmeijer *et al.* conducted the multicentre RCT named HAMLET (Hemicraniectomy After MCA infarction with Life-threatening [O]Edema Trial) performed in the Netherlands, the protocol of which was published in *Trials* in 2006.

There were no significant differences in the outcome measures between the three trials at the time of the pooled analysis and following results were found. The ARR for mortality at 12 months was 51.2%. Seventy-five percent of survivors receiving medical care had a 'favourable' outcome (mRS <4) vs. 55% of survivors who received surgery. Forty-five percent of survivors who had surgery had an mRS of 4 vs. 8% of those who received medical care.

Conclusions

DECIMAL: Decompressive surgery improves survival in young patients with MMI but with an increased number of patients with mRS.

DESTINY: Pooled analysis – Early decompressive surgery for MMI reduces mortality and increases the number of patients with a favourable functional outcome.

HAMLET: Surgical decompression within 48 hours of the onset of symptomatic MCA infarction did not improve functional outcomes compared to medical treatment.

The authors of the HAMLET trial updated the pooled analysis of the DESTINY/ DECIMAL/HAMLET trials and reported a benefit of surgery for those operated on within 48 hours of the onset of stroke symptoms. However, no conclusions can be drawn about those patients operated on after this time period. Age has certainly got an important effect on outcome as it appears that the mortality even with surgery for patients with MMI aged >50 years is more than twice that of patients aged <50 years.

Study references

Vahedi K, Vicaut E, Mateo J, Kurtz A, Orabi M, Guichard JP, Boutron C, Couvreur G, Rouanet F, Touzé E, Guillon B, Carpentier A, Yelnik A, George B, Payen D, Bousser MG, for the DECIMAL Investigators. Sequential-design, multicenter, randomised, controlled trial of early decompressive craniectomy in malignant middle cerebral artery infarction (DECIMAL trial). *Stroke* 2007; *38*: 2506–2517.

Jüttler E, Schwab S, Schmiedek P, Unterberg A, Hennerici M, Woitzik J, Witte S, Jenetzky E, Hacke W; DESTINY Study Group. Decompressive Surgery for the Treatment of Malignant Infarction of the Middle Cerebral Artery (DESTINY): a randomized, controlled trial. *Stroke* 2007 Sep; *38(9)*: 2518–2525. DOI: 10.1161/STROKEAHA.107.485649. Epub 2007 Aug 9. PMID: 17690310.

Hofmeijer J, Amelink GJ, Algra A, van Gijn J, Macleod MR, Kappelle LJ, van der Worp HB; HAMLET Investigators. Hemicraniectomy after middle cerebral artery infarction with life threatening edema trial (HAMLET). Protocol for a randomised controlled trial of decompressive surgery in space-occupying hemispheric infarction. *Trials* 2006; *7*: 29.

Pooled Analysis of DECIMAL, DESTINY, and HAMLET Trials Vahedi, K, Hofmeijer J, Juettler E, Vicaut E, George B, Algra A, Amelink GJ, Schmiedeck P, Schwab S, Rothwell PM, Bousser MG, van der Worp HB, Hacke W, for the DECIMAL, DESTINY and HAMLET Investigators. Early decompressive surgery in malignant infarction of the middle cerebral artery: a pooled analysis of three randomised trials. *Lancet Neurol* 2007; *6*: 215–222.

Other important publications for stroke

Aaslid R, Markwalder TM, Nornes H. Noninvasive transcranial Doppler ultrasound recording of flow velocity in basal cerebral arteries. *J Neurosurg* 1981; *57(6)*: 769–774.

Barnett HJ, Taylor DW, Eliasziw M, *et al*. Benefit of carotid endarterectomy in patients with symptomatic moderate or severe stenosis. North American Symptomatic Carotid Endarterectomy Trial Collaborators.*N Engl J Med* 1998; *339(20)*: 1415–1425.

European Carotid Surgery Trialists Collaboration Group. Randomised trial of endarterectomy for recently symptomatic carotid stenosis: final results of the MRC European Carotid Surgery Trial (ECST). *Lancet* 1998; *351(9113)*: 1379–1387.

Executive Committee for the Asymptomatic Carotid Atherosclerosis Study. Endarterectomy for asymptomatic carotid artery stenosis. *JAMA* 1995; *273(18)*: 1421–1428.

Ferguson GG, Eliasziw M, Barr HW, *et al*. The North American Symptomatic Carotid Endarterectomy Trial: surgical results in 1415 patients. *Stroke* 1999; *30(9)*: 1751–1758.

Kirollos RW, Tyagi AK, Ross SA, *et al*. Management of spontaneous cerebellar hematomas: a prospective treatment protocol. *Neurosurgery* 2001; *49(6)*: 1378–1386; discussion 1386–1387.

Mayberg MR, Wilson SE, Yatsu F, *et al*. Carotid endarterectomy and prevention of cerebral ischemia in symptomatic carotid stenosis. Veterans Affairs Cooperative Studies Program 309 Trialist Group. *JAMA* 1991; *266(23)*: 3289–3294.

North American Symptomatic Carotid Endarterectomy Trial Collaborators. Beneficial effect of carotid endarterectomy in symptomatic patients with high-grade carotid stenosis. *N Engl J Med* 1991; *325(7)*: 445–453.

Neuro-oncology

Extent of resection of low-grade gliomas

McGirt *et al.* published "Extent of surgical resection is independently associated with survival in patients with hemispheric low-grade glioma" in *Neurosurgery* in 2008. This retrospective study was carried out in Baltimore, Maryland, United States, with the analysis of patients who underwent resection low-grade glioma (LGG) at the Johns Hopkins Department of Neurosurgery between 1996 and 2007.

Overall survival (OS) and progression-free survival (PFS) in the Gross Total Resection group were 15 years and 7 years and OS and PFS were 7 years and 3.5 years. Even though there is a trend towards a better outcome, it was not statistically significant. The authors concluded that a greater extent of resection improves outcome for patients with low-grade glioma and should be safely attempted when not limited by eloquent cortex.

Study reference

McGirt MJ, Chaichana KL, Attenello FJ, Weingart JD, Than K, Burger P, Olivi AO, Brem H, Quinones-Hinojosa A. Extent of surgical resection is independently associated with survival in patients with hemispheric low-grade glioma. *Neurosurgery* 2008; *63*: 700–708.

Other important publications from neuro-oncology

Buckner JC, Shaw EG, Pugh SL. Radiation plus procarbazine, CCNU, and vincristine in low-grade glioma. *NEJM* 2016; *374*: 1344–1355.

Daumas-Duport C, Scheithauer B, O'Fallon J, et al. Grading of astrocytomas. A simple and reproducible method. *Cancer* 1988; *62(10)*: 2152–2165.

Hegi ME, Diserens AC, Gorlia T, et al. MGMT gene silencing and benefit from temozolomide in glioblastoma. *N Engl J Med* 2005; *352(10)*: 997–1003.

Keles GE, Lamborn KR, Berger MS. Low-grade hemispheric gliomas in adults: a critical review of extent of resection as a factor influencing outcome. *J Neurosurg* 2001; *95(5)*: 735–745.

Lacroix M, Abi-Said D, Fourney DR, et al. A multivariate analysis of 416 patients with glioblastoma multiforme: prognosis, extent of resection, and survival. *J Neurosurg* 2001; *95(2)*: 190–198

Lagerwaard FJ, Levendag PC, Nowak PJ, et al. Identification of prognostic factors in patients with brain metastases: a review of 1292 patients. *Int J Radiat Oncol Biol Phys* 1999; *43(4)*: 795–803.

Louis DN, Ohgaki H, Wiestler OD, et al. The 2007 WHO classification of tumours of the central nervous system. *Acta Neuropathol* 2007; *114(2)*: 97–109.

Patchell RA, Tibbs PA, Walsh JW, et al. A randomized trial of surgery in the treatment of single metastases to the brain. *N Engl J Med* 1990; *322(8)*: 494–500.

Simpson D. The recurrence of intracranial meningiomas after surgical treatment. *J Neurol Neurosurg Psychiatry* 1957; *20(1)*: 22–39.

Stummer W, Pichlmeier U, Meinel T, et al. (for the ALA-Glioma Study Group). Fluorescence-guided surgery with 5-aminolevulinic acid for resection of malignant glioma: a randomised controlled multicentre phase III trial. *Lancet Oncol* 2006; *7(5)*: 392–401.

Stupp R, Mason WP, Bent MJ, et al. Radiotherapy plus concomitant and adjuvant temozolomide for glioblastoma. *N Engl J Med* 2005; *352*: 987–996.

Walker MD, Alexander E Jr, Hunt WE, et al. Evaluation of BCNU and/or radiotherapy in the treatment of anaplastic gliomas. A cooperative clinical trial. *J Neurosurg* 1978; *49(3)*: 333–343.

Walker MD, Green SB, Byar DP, et al. Randomized comparisons of radiotherapy and nitro-soureas for the treatment of malignant glioma after surgery. N Engl J Med 1980; 303(23): 1323–1329.

Yaşargil MG, Kadri PA, Yaşargil DC. Microsurgery for malignant gliomas. J Neurooncol 2004; 69(1–3): 67–81.

Yung WK, Albright RE, Olson J, et al. A phase II study of temozolomide vs. procarbazine in patients with glioblastoma multiforme at first relapse. Br J Cancer 2000; 83: 588–593.

Spinal surgery

Steroids in spinal cord injury

The National Acute Spinal Cord Injury Study (NASCIS) is the largest study investigating the effects of the steroid methylprednisolone (MePred) in acute spinal cord injury (ASCI). There have been three parts to the study that are referred to as NASCIS I, NASCIS II and NASCIS III. These studies were carried out in the United States in the 1980s and 1990s.

In NASCIS I, the low-dose regimen (loading dose of MePred was 100 mg followed by 25 mg 6 hourly for 10 days) was compared with the moderate-dose regimen (1000 mg bolus followed by 250 mg 6 hourly for 10 days).

In NASCIS II, MePred was given as an intravenous bolus of 30 mg/kg followed by 5.4 mg/kg for 23 hours and was compared with placebo, and early vs. late treatment with steroid was compared.

In NASCIS III, MePred bolus and maintenance infusions were given as per NASCIS II except continued for a further 23 or 47 hours. NASCIS III also looked at ultra-early (<3 hours) vs. early (3–8 hours) administration of MePred.

NASCIS I study revealed that there was no difference between low- and moderate dose MePred. If given within 8 hours, moderate-dose MePred showed a trend towards a better outcome.

NASCIS II study revealed patients who received MePred within 8 hours of injury had a statistically significant improvement in motor and sensory function.

NASCIS III study results showed no statistically significant benefit of MePred when continued treatment for 48 hours. Also, there was no statistically significant benefit for ultra-early administration of MePred.

The authors concluded from three studies that MePred improves the outcome of ASCI if given within 8 hours of injury. However, the results remain controversial, and there is no guideline or recommendations regarding the use of steroids in ASCI. The use of MePred is, therefore, still a treatment choice available to the managing surgeon, and more surgeons are abandoning it.

Study references

Bracken MB, Collings WF, Freeman DF, Shepard MJ, Wagner FW, Silten RM, Hellenbrand KG, Ransohoff J, Hunt WE, Perot PL Jr, Grossman RG, Green BA, Eisenberg HM, Rifkinson N, Goodman JH, Meagher JN, Fischer B, Clifton GL, Flamm ES, Rawe SE. Efficacy of methylprednisolone in acute spinal cord injury. JAMA 1984; 251: 45–52.

Bracken MB, Shepard MJ, Hellenbrand KG, Collins WF, Leo LS, Freeman DF, Wagner FC, Flamm ES, Eisenberg HM, Goodman JH, Perot PL Jr, Green BA, Grossman RG, Meagher JN, Young W, Fischer B, Clifton GL, Hunt WE, Rifkinson N. Methylprednisolone and neurological function 1 year after spinal cord injury. Results of the National Acute Spinal Cord Injury Study. J Neurosurg 1985; 63: 704–713.

Bracken MB, Shepard MJ, Collins WF, Holford TR, Young W, Baskin DS, Eisenberg HM, Flamm E, Leo-Summers L, Maroon J, Marshall LF, Perot PL Jr, Piepmeier J, Sonntag VKH, Wagner FC, Wilberger JE, Winn HR. A randomized, controlled trial of methylprednisolone or naloxone in the treatment of acute spinal-cord injury. Results of the Second National Acute Spinal Cord Injury Study. N Engl J Med 1990; 322: 1405–1411.

Bracken MB, Shepard MJ, Holford TR, Leo-Summers L, Aldrich EF, Fazl M, Fehlings M, Herr DL, Hitchon PW, Marshall LF, Nockels RP, Pascale V, Perot PL Jr, Piepmeier J, Sonntag VK, Wagner F, Wilberger JE, Winn HR, Young W. Administration of methylprednisolone for 24 or 48 hours or tirilazad mesylate for 48 hours in the treatment of acute spinal cord injury. Results of the Third National Acute Spinal Cord Injury Randomized Controlled Trial. National Acute Spinal Cord Injury Study. JAMA 1997; 277: 1597–1604.

Steroid use in metastatic spinal cord compression

Sorensen *et al.* conducted a blinded RCT of high-dose dexamethasone as an adjunct to radiotherapy in patients with metastatic spinal cord compression (MESCC) from solid tumours was carried out between 1987 and 1989 in Copenhagen, Denmark and published "Effect of high-dose dexamethasone in carcinomatous MESCC treated with radiotherapy: a randomized trial" in the *European Journal of Cancer* in 1994.

In this trial, patients with clinical and radiological evidence of MESCC were included and patients with lymphoma, surgical decompression, previous epidural metastases, meningeal carcinomatosis and peptic ulcers were excluded. Dexamethasone was administered as an IV bolus of 96 mg followed by an oral dose of 96 mg for 3 days.

No difference was noted in survival between the two groups. Side effects were noted in 11% of the dexamethasone-treated patients. A subgroup analysis of patients with breast cancer showed that 94% of patients receiving dexamethasone achieved a successful result compared to 69% receiving no steroids. This result was not statistically significant.

At 3 months, 81% patients on dexamethasone had a return of gait function, in comparison to 63% patients without steroid. This result was also not statistically significant. At 6 months, the percentage of ambulatory patients was 59% who were on steroid and 33% who were not on steroids ($p = 0.05$). Although the benefit reached only borderline statistical significance, the authors concluded that steroids should be used as an adjunct in malignant cord compression. This study established the role of steroids, and the practice is not to administer steroids routinely to all patients with MESCC.

Study reference

Sorensen PS, Helwig-Larson S, Mouridesen H, Hansen HH. Effect of high-dose dexamethasone in carcinomatous metastatic spinal cord compression treated with radiotherapy: a randomized trial. Eur J Cancer 1994; 30A: 22–27.

Timing of surgery for acute spinal cord injury

Vaccaro *et al.* conducted an RCT between early surgery vs. late surgery for the cervical spinal cord for ASCI at the Regional Spinal Cord Injury Center of Delaware Valley from 1992 to 1995 and published "Neurologic outcome of early versus later surgery for cervical cord injury" in *Spine* in 1997.

Inclusion criteria were age 15–75 years; neurological impairment A–D on American Spinal Injury Association (ASIA) scale; neurological level C3–T1; admission within 48 hours of injury and radiological evidence of cord compression. Exclusion criteria were patients having other injuries preventing neurological evaluation or surgery; coexisting spinal cord disease and worsening neurology due to blood, disc or bony fragments within the canal. Early surgery was regarded as those <72 hours from injury and late surgery was >5 days from injury. Mean time to surgery was 1.8 days in the early group and 16.8 days in the late group. No significant difference was noted in the neurological or functional outcomes between the two groups or in the length of hospital stay. It was concluded that there is no benefit between surgery within 72 hours of injury and delayed surgery in cervical spinal cord injury.

This study was criticized as it included only cases of cervical cord injury and the mean length of time to early surgery, which was 1.8 days, may not be early enough. Earlier surgery within 8 or 12 hours of injury may have beneficial effect.

Study reference

Vaccaro AR, Daugherty RJ, Sheehan J, Sheehan TP, Dante SJ, Cotle JM, Balsderston, RA, Herbison GJ, Northup BE. Neurologic outcome of early versus later surgery for cervical cord injury. *Spine* 1997; *22*: 2609–2613.

Decompressive surgery for spinal metastasis

Bluegrass Neuro-Oncology Consortium in the United States conducted this multi-institutional study which is the largest randomized study which evaluated the role of decompressive surgery in the management of MESCC. Patchell *et al.* published the result of the study – "Direct decompressive surgical resection in the treatment of spinal cord compression caused by metastatic cancer: a randomised trial" in *Lancet* in 2005.

In this study, surgery plus radiotherapy was compared with radiotherapy alone. MESCC was defined radiologically as displacement of the spinal cord by an epidural mass. Inclusion criteria were age >18 years; at least one neurological sign; tissue diagnosis of non-CNS tumour and prognosis >3 months. Exclusion criteria were paraplegia >48 hours; radiosensitive tumour (lymphomas, leukaemia, multiple myeloma, germ cell tumour); previous MESCC.

Surgery followed by the radiotherapy group was clearly superior to help the patients walk or recover the ability to walk or retain the ability to walk and the comparison with the radiotherapy-only group show statistically significant difference. Therefore, the trial was stopped early from interim analysis. Patients in the surgery group also did significantly better in all secondary outcomes like continence, functional scores, muscle strength and less steroid use.

The authors concluded that surgical decompression with radiotherapy is superior to radiotherapy alone in MESCC.

Study reference

Patchell RA, Tibbs PA, Regine WF, Payne R, Saris S, Kryscio RJ, Mohiuddin M, Young B. Direct decompressive surgical resection in the treatment of spinal cord compression caused by metastatic cancer: a randomised trial. *Lancet* 2005 Aug 20–26; *366(9486)*: 643–8. DOI: 10.1016/S0140-6736(05)66954-1. PMID: 16112300.

Spine Patient Outcomes Research Trial (SPORT) study

Weinstein *et al.* conducted SPORT study to evaluate surgery vs. conservative management for prolapsed lumbar disc in the United States between 2000 and 2004 and published "Surgical vs nonoperative treatment of lumbar disk herniation: the Spine Patient Outcomes Research Trial (SPORT): a randomised trial" in *JAMA* in 2006.

The results showed that at 3 months, patients who chose surgery had greater improvement in the primary outcome measures of bodily pain, physical function and Oswestry Disability Index. These differences narrowed somewhat at 2 years. The authors concluded that patients received benefit from both surgery and conservative management, but no conclusions regarding the superiority of either can be made on an intention-to-treat analysis.

There is a criticism that SPORT study is hampered because of the large number of crossovers between treatment groups. But the supporters of the trial argue that this reflects the reality of spinal practice and is the only way in which a trial for this condition can be carried out.

Study reference

Weinstein JN, Tosteson TD, Lurie JD, Tosteson ANA, Hnascom B, Skinner JS, Abdu WA, Hilibrand AS, Boden SD, Deyo RA. Surgical vs nonoperative treatment of lumbar disk herniation: the Spine Patient Outcomes Research Trial (SPORT): a randomised trial. *JAMA* 2006; 296: 2441–2450.

Surgery in cauda equina syndrome (CES)

Todd looked at patients in the literature who had been operated on within 24 or 48 hours from the onset of CES. He accomplished a meta-analysis from six clinical studies that report the effect of 'early'/'late' decompression following CES. The timing of surgery was the only one input variable and the recovery of sphincter function was the only output variable analysed in the paper.

Meta-analysis demonstrates that patients treated <24 hours following the onset of CES are more likely to benefit from surgery in terms of recovery of bladder function than those treated >24 hours ($p = 0.03$). The patients who are operated within 48 hours after the onset of CES are more likely to benefit from surgery than those treated after 48 hours ($p = 0.005$). The timing of surgery following CES probably does influence outcome.

Study reference

Todd NV. Cauda equina syndrome: the timing of surgery probably does influence outcome. *Br J Neurosurg* 2005; *19*: 301–306.

Other important publications from spinal neurosurgery

Forsth P, Olafsson G, Carlsson T. A randomised, control trial of fusion surgery for lumbar spinal stenosis. *NEJM* 2016; *374(15)*: 1413–1423.

Legaye J, Duval-Beaupère G, Hecquet J, *et al*. Pelvic incidence: a fundamental pelvic parameter for three-dimensional regulation of spinal sagittal curves. *Eur Spine J* 1998; *7(2)*: 99–103.

Lenke LG, Betz RR, Harmes J, *et al*. Adolescent idiopathic scoliosis: a new classification to determine extent of spinal arthrodesis. *J Bone Joint Surg Am* 2001; *83(8)*: 1169–1181.

Pearson AM, Lurie JD, Tosteson TD. Who should undergo surgery for degenerative spondylolisthesis. Treatment and effect predictors in SPORT. *Spine* 2013; *38*:1799–1811.

Weinstein JN, Lurie JD, Tosteson TD, *et al*. Surgical versus nonsurgical therapy for lumbar spinal stenosis. *N Engl J Med* 2008; *358(8)*: 794–810.

Weinstein JN, Lurie JD, Tosteson TD, *et al*. Surgical versus nonsurgical treatment for lumbar degenerative spondylolisthesis. *N Engl J Med* 2007; *356*: 2257–2270.

Wilby MJ, Best A, Wood E. Surgical microdiscectomy versus transforaminal epidural steroid injection in patients with sciatica secondary to herniated lumbar disc (NERVES): a phase 3, multicentre, open-label, randomised controlled trial and economic evaluation. *Lancet Rheumatology* 2021; *3(5)*: E347–356.

Neurosurgical treatment of trigeminal neuralgia

Microvascular decompression for trigeminal neuralgia

Janetta's group in 1996 published the results of a series of 1185 patients from the Presbyterian-University Hospital in Pittsburgh, Pennsylvania, United States, undergoing microvascular decompression (MVD) between 1972 and 1991, and the long-term outcome of MVD for trigeminal neuralgia (TN) was established.

Excellent outcome was achieved in 82% of patients in the immediate post-operative period. The number tapered to 75% in 1 year and further reduced to 64% in 10 years. Good outcome was reported in 16% in the immediate post-operative period, 9% in 1 year and 4% in 10 years. When repeat surgery was included, excellent outcomes were achieved in 80% of patients at 1 year and 70% of patients at 10 years.

The commonest offending vessel was the superior cerebellar artery (75%). Venous compression was seen in 68%. Though complications were uncommon, CSF leak, hearing loss and facial numbness were noted as the most frequent ones.

Recurrence of the pain was found at the rate of <2% at 5 years and <1% at 10 years. Risk factors for recurrence included lack of immediate post-operative relief, female sex, venous compression and pre-operative symptoms of >8 years' duration.

The authors concluded that MVD for TN is safe and has a high rate of long-term success rate.

Study references

Barker FG, Janetta PJ, Bissonette DJ, PAC, Larkins MV, Jho HD. The long-term outcome of microvascular decompression for trigeminal neuralgia. *N Engl J Med* 1996; *334*: 1077–1083.

Janetta PJ. Arterial compression of the trigeminal nerve at the pons in patients with trigeminal neuralgia. *J Neurosurgery* 1976; *26*: 159–162.

Other landmark publications from the skull base

Bills DC, Meyer FB, Laws ER Jr, et al. A retrospective analysis of pituitary apoplexy. *Neurosurgery* 1993; *33(4)*: 602–608; discussion 608–609.

Cappabianca P, Cavallo LM, de Divitiis E. Endoscopic endonasal transsphenoidal surgery. *Neurosurgery* 2004; *55(4)*: 933–940; discussion 940–941.

Hardy DG, Rhoton AL. Microsurgical relationships of the superior cerebellar artery and the trigeminal nerve. *J Neurosurg* 1978; *49(5)*: 669–678.

House JW, Brackmann DE. Facial nerve grading system. *Otolaryngol Head Neck Surg* 1985; *93(2)*: 146–147.

Jannetta PJ. Arterial compression of the trigeminal nerve at the pons in patients with trigeminal neuralgia. *J Neurosurg* 1967; *26(1)*: 159–162.

National Institutes of Health Consensus Development Conference. *Acoustic Neuroma: Consensus statement*. NIH Consens Dev Conf Consens Statement, Vol. 9. 1991.

Rhoton AL. The cerebellopontine angle and posterior fossa cranial nerves by the retrosigmoid approach. *Neurosurgery* 2000; *47(3 Suppl)*: S93–129.

Rhoton AL. Microsurgical anatomy of the brainstem surface facing an acoustic neuroma. *Surg Neurol* 1986; *25*: 326–339.

Ross DA, Wilson CB. Results of transsphenoidal microsurgery for growth hormone-secreting pituitary adenoma in a series of 214 patients. *J Neurosurg* 1998; *68(6)*: 854–867.

Rutherford SA, King AT. Vestibular schwannoma management: what is the "best" option? *Br J Neurosurg* 2005; *19(4)*: 309–316.

Hydrocephalus

BASICS trial

Mallucci *et al.* carried out this parallel, multicentre, single-blind, RCT to evaluate the cost effectiveness of the antibiotic-impregnated shunts, silver shunts and standard shunts. They included patients with hydrocephalus of any aetiology undergoing insertion of their first ventriculoperitoneal shunt irrespective of age at 21 regional adult and paediatric neurosurgery centres in the UK and Ireland. Patients were randomly assigned to receive standard shunts, antibiotic-impregnated (0·15% clindamycin and 0·054% rifampicin) or silver-impregnated shunts. In 22 months follow-up, 2% patients of the antibiotic-impregnated shunt group and 6% patients of both silver-impregnated shunt group and standard shunt group needed revision of the shunts for infection. This was statistically significant to favour the antibiotic-impregnated shunts.

The authors concluded that this trial provides evidence to support the adoption of antibiotic shunts in UK patients who are having their first ventriculoperitoneal shunt insertion. This practice will benefit patients of all ages by reducing the risk and harm of shunt infection.

Study reference

Mallucci CL, Jenkinson MD, Conroy EJ, Hartley JC, Brown M, Dalton J, Kearns T, Moitt T, Griffiths MJ, Culeddu G, Solomon T, Hughes D, Gamble C; BASICS Study Collaborators. Antibiotic or silver versus standard ventriculoperitoneal shunts (BASICS): a multi-centre, single-blinded, randomised trial and economic evaluation. *Lancet* 2019 Oct 26; *394(10208)*: 1530–1539. DOI: 10.1016/S0140-6736(19)31603-4. Epub 2019 Sep 12. Erratum in: *Lancet* 2019 Sep 18; Erratum in: *Lancet* 2020 Jun 13; *395(10240)*: 1834. PMID: 31522843; PMCID: PMC6999649.

Other important publications for hydrocephalus

Adams RD, Fisher CM, Hakim S, *et al*. Symptomatic occult hydrocephalus with "normal" cerebrospinal-fluid pressure. A treatable syndrome. *N Engl J Med* 1965; *273*: 117–126.

Brodbelt A, Stoodley M. CSF pathways: a review. *Br J Neurosurg* 2007; *21(5)*: 510–520.

Important publications from functional neurosurgery

Benabid AL, Pollak P, Gao D, *et al*. Chronic electrical stimulation of the ventralis intermedius nucleus of the thalamus as a treatment of movement disorders. *J Neurosurg* 1996; *84(2)*: 203–214.

Benabid AL, Pollak P, Louveau A, *et al*. Combined (thalamotomy and stimulation) stereotactic surgery of the VIM thalamic nucleus for bilateral Parkinson disease. *Appl Neurophysiol* 1987; *50(1-6)*: 344–346.

Coubes P, Roubertie A, Vayssiere N, *et al*. Treatment of DYT1-generalised dystonia by stimu-lation of the internal globus pallidus. *Lancet* 2000; *355(9222)*: 2220–2221.

Leksell L. The stereotaxic method and radiosurgery of the brain. *Acta Chir Scand* 1951; *102(4)*: 316–319.

Limousin P, Pollak P, Benazzouz A, *et al*. Bilateral subthalamic nucleus stimulation for severe Parkinson's disease. *Mov Disord* 1995; *10(5)*: 672–674.

May A, Bahra A, Büchel C, *et al*. Hypothalamic activation in cluster headache attacks. *Lancet* 1998; *352(9124)*: 275–278.

Wiebe S, Blume WT, Girvin JP, *et al*. (Effectiveness and Efficiency of Surgery for Temporal Lobe Epilepsy Study Group). A randomized, controlled trial of surgery for temporal lobe epilepsy. *N Engl J Med* 2001; *345(5)*: 311–318.

Other

Collen JF, Jackson JL, Shorr AF *et al*. Prevention of venous thromboembolism in neurosur-gery: a metaanalysis. *Chest* 2008; *134*: 237–249.

8 | Key Terms

Arachnoid cyst – cerebrospinal fluid covered by arachnoid cells and collagen. It is benign and occurs in the cerebrospinal axis in relation to the arachnoid membrane. It does not communicate with the ventricular system.

Athetosis – a continuous stream of slow writhing movements, typically of the hands and feet, often caused by damage to the corpus striatum.

Chiari malformation – a condition characterized by a downward displacement of the cerebellar tonsils and the medulla through the foramen magnum sometimes causing obstructive hydrocephalus as a result of obstruction of cerebral spinal fluid (CSF) outflow.

- Chiari Type 0 is the absence of the tonsils below the foramen magnum. It includes the presence of symptoms and a syrinx in the spinal cord. Controversial.
- Chiari Type 1 is the most common type, is due to impaired CSF circulation through the foramen magnum. Commonly, the cerebral tonsillar herniation is >5 mm below the foramen magnum. In 30–70%, there is an associated syringomyelia.
- Chiari Type 2, Arnold–Chiari malformation, results in caudally dislocated cervicomedullary junction, pons, fourth ventricle and medulla. The cerebellar tonsils are located at or below the foramen magnum. Usually associated with a myelomeningocele.
- Chiari Type 3 is the most severe form, results in the displacement of the posterior fossa structures, with cerebellum herniation through the foramen magnum into cervical canal. It is often associated with a high cervical or suboccipital encephalomeningocele.
- Chiari Type 4 is cerebellar hypoplasia without cerebellar herniation.

Table 8.1 Chiari malformation Type 1 and 2

	Type 1	Type 2
Age of presentation	Young adult	Child
Usual presentation	Neck pain/headaches	Hydrocephalus/respiratory distress
Caudal dislocation of medulla	–	+
Caudal dislocation into the cervical canal	Tonsils	Inferior vermis, medulla, 4th ventricle
Hydrocephalus	–	+
Medullary 'kink'	–	+ (50%)
Course of upper cranial nerves	Normal	Cephalad

DOI: 10.1201/9781003254379-8

Chorea – an involuntary movement disorder characterized by brief, irregular contractions that are not repetitive or rhythmic but appear to flow from one muscle to the next.

Colloid cyst – a benign, epithelium-lined cyst believed to originate from the anterior part of the third ventricle. The cysts are believed to derive from either primitive neuroepithelium of the tela choroidea or from the endoderm. Because of its location, it can cause obstructive hydrocephalus and increased intracranial pressure (ICP).

Craniopharyngioma – a benign, epithelium-lined cyst believed to originate from the anterior margin of the sella turcica. It has benign histology and malignant behaviour.

- Embryogenetic theory suggests that the adamantinomatous type ('adamantinoma') arises from epithelial remnants of the involuted Rathke's pouch or the craniopharyngeal duct.
- Metaplastic theory suggests that the squamous papillary type results due to the metaplasia of residual squamous epithelium that arises from squamous cell nests normally found at the junction of the pituitary stalk and pars distalis.

Dermoid and epidermoid cysts – these are not true neoplasms but are inclusion cysts composed of ectodermal elements resulting from a developmental abnormality. Centrally, they contain desquamated epithelial keratin and lipid material. The external surface is smooth, lobulated and pearly in appearance. They are lined with stratified squamous epithelium and contain an outer connective tissue capsule. Cyst characteristics and location distinguish them.

- Dermoid tumours include other dermal elements (hair, teeth, follicles, sebaceous glands), and they are located near the midline. They are associated with other congenital anomalies in up to 50% of cases.
- Epidermoids are located laterally. They tend to be isolated lesions.

Dural arteriovenous fistula – an abnormal direct connection (fistula) between a meningeal artery and a meningeal vein or dural venous sinus. The Borden classification of dural arteriovenous malformations or fistulas is based on the venous drainage.

- Type I: dural arterial supply drains anterograde into venous sinus.
- Type II: dural arterial supply drains into venous sinus. High pressure in sinus results in both anterograde drainage and retrograde drainage via subarachnoid veins.
- Type III: dural arterial supply drains retrograde into subarachnoid veins.

Cortical venous drainage determines those with high risk or more malignant clinical course based on the effects of venous hypertension or intracranial haemorrhage. These factors also help determine the indication for intervention.

Ependymoma – a glial tumour that arises from ependymal cells lining the cerebral ventricles and the central canal of the spinal cord. In the paediatric population, it tends to be located intracranially (fourth ventricle). In the adult population, it tends to be located in the spine (WHO 2021).

Haemangioblastoma – a benign, highly vascular tumour that can occur in the brain and spine. It is composed of endothelial cells, pericytes and stromal cells. Most haemangioblastomas are single lesions. They can be associated with Von Hippel–Lindau disease (VHL; see below).

Diagnostic criteria of Von Hippel–Lindau disease (VHL)

Patients without a family history of VHL
- Two or more CNS haemangioblastomas
- One CNS haemangioblastoma and a visceral tumour (excluding epididymal or renal cysts)

Patients with a family history of VHL
- One CNS haemangioblastoma

  or

- Phaeochromocytoma

  or

- Clear cell renal carcinoma

Hemiballismus – a unilateral wild, large-amplitude flinging involuntary movement of the proximal part of the limbs, which results in postural imbalance. It is caused by a decrease in the activity of the subthalamic nucleus of the basal ganglia.

Hydromyelia – a fluid collection within the spinal cord lined by ependymal cells.

Idiopathic intracranial hypertension – a condition characterized by increased ICP without evidence of intracranial mass, infection, hydrocephalus or hypertensive encephalopathy.

Medulloblastoma – one of the family of primitive neuroectodermal tumours (PNETs). This tumour is the most common paediatric brain malignancy and the most common PNET. It usually arises in the roof of the fourth ventricle, which can lead to hydrocephalus. Brainstem invasion often limits complete surgical excision. A whole-spine MRI scan is required to assess for drop metastasis.

Meningioma – a tumour that arises from arachnoid cap cells of the arachnoid villi in the meninges.

An important change in the 5th Edition (2021) WHO classification of CNS tumours is that the identification of some histological subtypes (e.g. papillary meningiomas and rhabdoid meningiomas) is no longer sufficient to denote a higher grade.

Grade 2 criteria
- Increased mitotic figures: 4–19 in 10 consecutive high-power fields (HPFs)
- Brain invasion
- Chordoid or clear cell histological subtype
- Three or more of the following:
  - Increased cellularity
  - Prominent nucleoli
  - Necrosis

- Sheet-like growth
- Small cells with a high nuclear to cytoplasmic ratio

Grade 3 criteria
- Increased mitotic figures: ≥20 in 10 consecutive HPFs
- Homozygous deletion of CDKN2A/B
- Sarcoma or carcinoma or melanoma-like appearance
- TERT promoter mutation

Traditionally, the grade would be determined by subtype (see the table below). Subtype no longer defines the grade.

The WHO classification of meningiomas

Benign (Grade I) (90%)	Meningothelial, fibrous, transitional, psammomatous, angiomatous, microcystic, secretory, lymphoplasmacyte-rich, metaplastic
Atypical (Grade II) (7%)	Chordoid, clear cell, atypical
Anaplastic/malignant (Grade III) (2%)	Papillary, rhabdoid, anaplastic

Myoclonus – a brief, involuntary twitching of a muscle or a group of muscles.

Neuroenteric cyst – an intradural extramedullary cystic mass lined by gut endothelium.

Neurofibromatosis – an autosomal dominant disorder in which there is a risk of tumour formation in the brain. The disorder affects neural crest cells (e.g. Schwann cells, melanocytes and endoneurial fibroblasts). Cellular elements from these cell types proliferate throughout the body, forming tumours and disordered skin pigmentation. NF1 is due to a mutation in the NF1 gene (on chromosome 17) that allows the production of the protein neurofibromin. NF2 is due to a mutation in the NF2 gene (chromosome 22) that allows the production of a protein called merlin.

Diagnostic criteria of neurofibromatosis type I

1. ≥6 café au lait macules >5 mm in greatest diameter in prepubertal individuals and >15 mm in greatest diameter in postpubertal individuals

2. ≥2 neurofibromas of any type or >1 plexiform neurofibroma

3. Freckling in the axillary or inguinal regions

4. Optic glioma

5. ≥2 Lisch nodules (iris hamartomas)

6. A distinctive osseous lesion, such as sphenoid dysplasia or thinning of the long bone cortex, with or without pseudoarthrosis

7. A first-degree relative (parent, sibling or offspring) with NF-1 according to the above criteria

Diagnostic criteria of neurofibromatosis type II

1. Bilateral vestibular schwannomas (VS) OR family history of NF-2 1 unilateral VS
   OR
   Any 2 of meningioma, glioma, neurofibroma, schwannoma or posterior subcapsular lenticular opacities
   Additional criteria

2. Unilateral VS plus any two of meningioma, glioma, neurofibroma, schwannoma or posterior subcapsular opacities
   OR

3. Multiple meningioma (>2) plus unilateral VS OR any two of glioma, neurofibroma, schwannoma or cataract

Normal pressure hydrocephalus – a condition characterized by a triad of cognitive impairment, gait disturbance and urinary incontinence. ICP measurements are not usually elevated.

Pain – a physiological response to noxious stimuli (e.g. thermal, mechanical, chemical and trauma) that are damaging to the underlying tissues.

Papilloedema – optic disc swelling that is caused by increased ICP. Fundoscopy may reveal venous engorgement, loss of venous pulsation, haemorrhages, blurring of optic margins or elevation of the optic disc. On visual field examination, there may be an enlarged blind spot. Visual acuity is normal until papilloedema has become advanced.

Parkinson's disease – a neurological syndrome characterized by tremor (resting, 4–7/s), cogwheel rigidity and bradykinesia. Other signs include postural instability, micrographia, mask-like facies or a festinating gait. It is the result of degeneration of pigmented dopaminergic neurons of the pars compacta of the substantia nigra, resulting in reduced levels of dopamine in the neostriatum (e.g. caudate nucleus, putamen, globus pallidus).

Rathke's cleft cyst – a benign, epithelium-lined intrasellar cyst found on the pituitary gland, which occurs when Rathke's pouch does not develop properly.

Modified Frisén scale for grading papilloedema

STAGE 0 – Normal optic disc or not a disc but no oedema/swelling
A. Prominence of the retinal nerve fibre layer at the nasal, superior and inferior poles in inverse proportion to disc diameter
B. Radial nerve fibre layer striations, without tortuosity

STAGE I – Minimal
A. C-shaped halo that is subtle and greyish with a temporal gap; obscures underlying retinal details
B. Disruption of normal radial NFL arrangement striations
C. Temporal disc margin normal

STAGE II – Low degree
A. Circumferential halo
B. Elevation – nasal border
C. No major vessel obscuration

(Continued)

STAGE III – Moderate
A. Obscuration of one or more segments of major blood vessels leaving disc
B. Circumferential halo
C. Elevation – all borders
D. Halo – irregular outer fringe with finger-like extensions

STAGE IV – Marked
A. Total obscuration on the disc of a segment of a major blood vessel on the disc
B. Elevation – whole nerve head, including the cup
C. Border obscuration – complete
D. Halo – complete

STAGE V – Severe
A. Partial obscuration of all vessels on disc and total obscuration of at least one vessel on disc

Scales and scoring systems

General

- American Society of Anaesthesiologists' (ASA) classification.
- Glasgow Coma Scale (GCS).
- Glasgow Outcome Scale (GOS).
- Evan's ratio for hydrocephalus.
- Injury Severity Score (trauma).
- Karnofsky Performance Status Scale.
- Marshall's CT grading (trauma).
- Modified Rankin scale.
- Medical Research Council (MRC) grade for muscle power.

Functional

- Ashworth scores for spasticity.
- Engel's classification for epilepsy control following surgery.
- Parkinson's Disability Score.

Oncology

- Galassi classification for arachnoid cysts.
- Glasscock–Jackson glomus tympanicum classification.
- House–Brackmann grade of facial nerve function.
- MacDonald criteria for determining tumour progression.
- Simpson grades for extent of meningioma resection.

Spine

- American Spinal Injury Association (ASIA) scores.
- C1 fracture classification.
- C1 fracture – Rule of Spence.
- C2 hangman's fractures – Modified Effendi system.
- C2 odontoid fractures – Anderson and D'Alonzo classification.

- Basilar impression measurements: McRae's line, Chamberlain's line, McGregor's line, Wackenheim's clivus-canal line.
- Frankel grade.
- Nurick's classification for cervical myelopathy.
- Oswestry Disability Index.
- Ranawat classification for the neurological deficit.
- Meyerding classification for spondylolisthesis.
- Modic's classification for vertebral body marrow changes.
- Patchell criteria for metastatic spinal cord compression.
- Wiltse classification for spondylolisthesis.

Vascular

- Barrow classification for congestive cardiac failure (CCF).
- Burstein and Papile grading for neonatal intracranial haemorrhage.
- Congard or Borden classification for dual arteriovenous fistula (DAVF).
- Fisher grade for subarachnoid haemorrhage (SAH).
- Hunt and Hess classification of SAH.
- Modified Rankin Scale.
- PHASES score.
- Pollock and Flickinger score for arteriovenous malformation (AVM) grading for radiosurgery.
- Spetzler–Martin grade for AVMs.
- World Federation of Neurosurgeons (WFNS) classification for SAH.

Peripheral nerves

- Seddon and Sunderland's classification of peripheral nerve injury.

Seizure – an abnormal paroxysmal cerebral neuronal discharge that results in alteration of sensation, motor function, behaviour or consciousness.

Syringomyelia – the development of a fluid-filled cavity or syrinx within the spinal cord. Several theories have been put forth to explain the pathogenesis of syringomyelia.

- **Gardner's hydrodynamic theory** – results from a 'water hammer'-like transmission of pulsatile CSF pressure via a communication between the fourth ventricle and the central canal of the spinal cord through the obex. There are craniospinal pressure differentials in the setting of fourth ventricular outlet obstruction; these differentials favour cerebrospinal fluid shifts from the fourth ventricle of the brain through the central canal of the spinal cord.
- **William's theory (craniospinal pressure dissociation)** – due to a differential between ICP and spinal pressure caused by a valve-like action at the foramen magnum by the tonsils. An increase in subarachnoid fluid pressure from increased venous pressure during coughing or a valsalva manoeuvre is localized to the intracranial compartment.

- **Oldfield's theory** – it demonstrates that downward movement of the cerebellar tonsils during systole can be visualized with dynamic magnetic resonance imaging (MRI). This oscillation creates a piston effect in the spinal subarachnoid space that acts on the surface of the spinal cord and forces CSF through the perivascular and interstitial spaces into the syrinx, increasing intramedullary pressure. Signs and symptoms of neurological dysfunction that appear with distension of the syrinx are due to compression of long tracts, neurons and microcirculation. Symptoms referable to increased intramedullary pressure are potentially reversible by syrinx decompression.

	Resting tremor	Postural tremor	Action tremor
Description	Tremor when skeletal muscle is at rest.	Tremor when skeletal muscle is holding in one position against gravity.	Tremor when in process of voluntary contraction of muscle.
Physical exam test	Observe at rest Observe while asking the patient to do mental work (may increase).	Ask the patient to extend arms and hold.	Finger to the nose, rapid alternating movements or heel to the shin.
Examples	Parkinson's disease, Parkinsonian tremor (e.g. medications).	Essential tremor, increased physiologic tremor, Wilson's disease.	Cerebellar disease, multiple sclerosis, chronic alcohol abuse.

Tremor – an involuntary, rhythmical contraction of a muscle group and can be classified into resting, postural or action tremor. There can be an overlap between the categories listed in the figure.

Trigeminal neuralgia – a condition characterized by unilateral sudden paroxysmal facial pain described as sharp, lancinating or shooting and lasting a few seconds, confined to the distribution of one or more branches of the trigeminal nerve (V2 and V3). Often the pain is triggered by sensory stimuli (e.g. brushing teeth or hair, talking and eating). The pathophysiology is related to the ephaptic transmission in the trigeminal nerve from large-diameter partially demyelinated A fibres to thinly myelinated A-delta and C (nociceptive) fibres. Differential diagnosis includes atypical facial pain, cluster headache, dental disease, orbital disease, sinusitis, giant cell arteritis, herpes zoster, temporomandibular joint (TMJ) dysfunction and intracranial tumour (e.g. posterior fossa).

Vascular malformation – a blood vessel abnormality. The vascular lesion can be classified as follows:

- AVM is a mesh of abnormal blood vessels characterized by the absence of normal interposing capillaries with no intervening brain parenchyma. As a result, oxygenated blood drains directly into the venous channel.
- Cavernous malformation – it is an angiographically occult venous anomaly characterized by thin venous sinusoidal vessels with blood with no intervening brain matter. Its gross appearance resembles a mulberry.

- Capillary telangiectasia – it is an angiographically occult vascular anomaly characterized by slightly enlarged capillaries with low flow with normal intervening brain parenchyma. They may be associated with Osler–Weber–Rendu syndrome (hereditary haemorrhagic telangiectasia).
- Venous angioma – it is a tuft of abnormal medullary veins that converge into a large central trunk and drain into either a superficial or deep venous system. Intervening brain is present.

Vestibular schwannoma (acoustic schwannoma) – a benign intracranial extra-axial tumour that arises from the myelin-forming cells of the vestibulocochlear nerve.

Index

Note: Page references in *italics* denote figures and in **bold** tables.

Printed in the United States
by Baker & Taylor Publisher Services